ON THE
DOWN
LOW

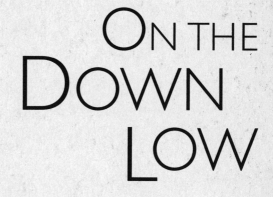

ON THE DOWN LOW

A Journey into the Lives of "Straight"
Black Men Who Sleep with Men

J. L. King
with Karen Hunter

BROADWAY BOOKS

NEW YORK

PRINTED IN THE UNITED STATES OF AMERICA

BROADWAY BOOKS and its logo, a letter B bisected on the diagonal, are
trademarks of Random House, Inc.

First edition published 2004

ISBN 0-7679-1398-1

I dedicate this book to all the women whose health has been jeopardized and emotional state compromised by men living on the DL, and to all women in general who may use this book as a protective guide. I also dedicate this book to men on the DL in hopes that looking in this mirror will be a catalyst to change.

Contents

Introduction:
The Journey to Self-Acceptance   ix

1   On the DL   1

2   "But I'm Not Gay!"   17

3   Was My Marriage a Lie?   29

4   She Can't Compete with Him   47

5   I Love the Ladies, Too   59

6   "Oh God!"   73

7   The Black Church   77

8   To Serve and Not Protect   85

9   The Criminal Justice System   93

10   Talking to Our Youth About Sex Is Key   105

11   Tops and Bottoms   119

12   The Signs   123

13 DL Behavior Types   135

14 Making Connections on the DL   153

15 A Need to Protect Ourselves and Others 161

16 No More Secrets   169

17 Your Opinion Matters   179

18 Women Still Want a Relationship   183

Acknowledgments   187

Introduction

The Journey to Self-Acceptance

When I first started on this journey as an "official" face of "Down Low" men, I knew that I was entering into something that would change my life forever. At first, I tried to do this work in denial, seeking to expose the behavior without exposing myself. I remember being interviewed by a reporter from *USA Today* and asking him not to use my last name in the story. I used the name "J. Louis" because I didn't want my identity known. And more importantly, I still wanted to be on the "DL." When I first accepted a speaking engagement in my hometown, I told my client to list me on the program as "J. Louis" and insisted that everyone call me by that name. I explained to her that I didn't want the word to get out that I was coming forward about my life. I was frightened that someone

I knew, or worse yet, a family member, would hear about me if I used my last name. Then I'd be busted, all of my secrets would be uncovered, and I wasn't ready for that. I was hiding and had convinced myself that I could get away with it. The need to hide my double lifestyle was so powerful that it overshadowed any common sense I had. As a result, my life was cloaked in lies.

I recall sharing with family and close friends, over Thanksgiving dinner, that I was speaking about HIV prevention in the black community. I kept my description vague. I didn't tell them that I was talking about my life, but talked about how the current trend of the virus was affecting our community. I lied.

After I mentioned that I would be featured in a BET interview, my sister-in-law asked me when the show was going to air. I told her that I didn't think the interview would air at all, explaining that the network had changed their minds. I lied again. I didn't want her or anyone else in my family tuning in to see me talking about my "DL" lifestyle. The fear of being exposed was more than I could bear.

I mistakenly believed that I could find safety in the lies. I even lied about my sexual orientation to the women who were my sexual partners. Even though I was traveling around the country, educating others on the dangers of DL behavior, I wasn't practicing what I was preaching. Even as the media began touting me as the "DL expert," the black man who was "telling health officials that they are missing the mark," I was still trying to hold on to my own DL behavior. I felt safe under the blanket of lies. I'd been there so long that coming out and standing in truth was something I didn't rush to do. Having grown weary from the secrecy and deceit that defined my existence, I prayed for guidance.

My heart was heavily burdened and I had no one to talk to about what was going on in my mind. Many times I wanted to resign from my role as a public activist and go back to being "me." I struggled enormously with the discrepancy between my public and private selves. I still wanted to hide from my past and wash it away as if it had never happened. At times I hated being alone because in those quiet moments I was forced to think about what I was doing and reckon with the contradictions I was living. My head pounded with questions: "Why do I have to speak out?" "What do I have to gain by coming forward?" Truth was calling but I wasn't ready to answer.

Still, over time, I eventually came to accept that there's no hiding from yourself. No matter how brilliant the performance put on for others, at the end of the day I still had to face myself.

Many DL men want to stop their duplicitous behavior and seek help, but they don't. They fear the ridicule and isolation commonly hurled their way by those who look upon them through a spirit of condemnation rather than through a spirit of compassion. The negative name calling, the jokes, the isolation, and the guilt are paralyzing. I know what's it like to have nowhere to turn. I didn't go to my pastor because I didn't trust him. When I talked to my fellow DL friends about the tremendous pull inside of me to come and share this message, they sought to discourage me. I felt that no one understood. There was no one to turn to until I met a strong sister whom I instantly connected with, Juliet Dorris-Williams. She offered an understanding ear as I poured out the inner turmoil I was experiencing. She listened without judgment and encouraged me to follow the directive of my heart. She asserted that even though I would be attacked, discredited, and disliked, I should stand in truth anyway for two reasons: I'd be helping others, and, in the end, it would make me a better man. I know now that I was led to her to receive that message and become bolstered up with enough courage to face my past, relinquish it, and move forward with my life.

When I reflect on the twenty-five years that I lived on the DL, it doesn't make me happy. I feel ashamed of my behavior and the impact it had on the people in my life. I want to call every woman and every man that I used solely for the fulfillment of my own personal desires and apologize. My mind is heavy with thoughts of the sisters who fell in love with me and gave their all because they believed me when I would look them in the eye and profess my love for them and promise my tomorrows to them. Even though I meant every word I said as I spoke it, I was so confused on the inside that I couldn't live up to being the man they hoped me to be. My heart is heavy with the memory of leaving the arms of these women, happily exhaling, to go and have sex with men. My soul is heavy with remembrances of all of the social gatherings I attended with my girlfriends, acting as a perfect gentleman while secretly trying to hook up with other men at these events. Sometimes the men were their brothers or other family members. Being untrue to myself resulted in my being untrue to everyone else. I hate what I did and the pain my behavior caused for others.

I am a new man. Through the transforming power of God's love, I am a different person. I realize that I was wrong to try to make choices for the women who were in my life. By denying them the truth, I denied them the respect, honor, and freedom of choice they were rightfully due.

Now that I'm living in the resurrection of God's love I am at peace. I know and accept who I am. I am fully aware that a relationship is a sacred trust that can only be sustained through openness and honesty. I know the importance of being true to myself and honestly representing myself to others. Self-acceptance is necessary before any hope of being accepted by others can be realized. That's one of the biggest lessons I've learned on this journey. Now, when I have conversations with friends about the transformation of my life, it feels good. My self-acceptance is clear to all who meet me.

Often I'm asked why I'm telling my story, what made me come clean? I can't take credit for stepping out on my own. This work was ordained by God. I was seeking guidance and clarity about my life's purpose, and this work is the answer to my prayers. Growing up, I heard "Be careful what you pray for because you just might get it." Now I know it's true because that's exactly what happened to me. I wanted to know God's purpose for my life, and it has been revealed to me. I know that I'm on the right path because it's been confirmed to me in many ways. From day one, everything and everyone I've needed to carry this message forth has appeared with no prompting from me except prayer. I had no connections to help me get invited to speak. Nor did I have a public relations professional promoting my message to the media. Seemingly, out of nowhere the speaking engagements and media interviews found their way to me.

This work is also a testament to my love for the women who are and have been a part of my life. I've always had a close relationship with my daughter, who is now an adult pursuing her passion as a teacher. On the day she was born, she captured my heart and she's kept it ever since. Like most fathers, I've always been protective of my baby girl. When she was in high school, I didn't want her to date, but she did. I knew that one day she would go off to college to expand her world and I wouldn't be around to protect her. Still, I didn't think she could meet a brother who lived as I did during that time. I was so preoccupied with satisfying my own desires that I failed to see that my beloved baby girl could be subjected to the same dishonest behavior that I was guilty of at that time. Why do I do this work? So that my daughter and other young women will not have to experience the fallout of dealing with a man who isn't honest with them.

I do this work because I still love my ex-wife, the mother of my children. In high school, she was more than just my girlfriend. After we married, she was more than a wife. She was my best friend, confidante, and running partner. It's difficult for me to fathom how I lied to her, but I did. I walked in the house, after sexual encounters with men, as if nothing had happened. I didn't think of her life, her feelings, and her future. She suffered greatly when she found out. It took her years to trust men, and I believe that even today she still hurts from the experience. I can see it in her eyes when we are together, and I hear it in her voice when we speak. Though it's been more than twenty years since we were together, I don't think she's gotten over it. I know that I haven't. I'm still dealing with what I did to her, the pain I caused, and my inability to erase the pieces of our past that hurt her. If I could, I'd release her from the burden of her hurt and disappointment with me, leaving her with only the memory of the love that we shared. My double life was a fallacy, but our love was real.

I do this work for all of the women who have loved me and who deserved the truth from me during a time that I was unable to give it. I pray that in some small measure, my words and my life will be a source of comfort and restoration for them. And, finally, I do this work for every man who is lost in his own lies, living in the dungeon of deceit. Through the pages of this book, I pray that they find the strength and courage to rise up and become the men that our women deserve, that our community needs, and that God intended them to be.

ON THE
DOWN
LOW

ON THE DL

I spotted this brother from my pew, ten rows back. His broad shoulders seemed to take up two seats. His physique was not burly, but the definition of his muscles was noticeable even through his light wool suit. His face was striking. He was a light-skinned brother who wore his curly hair cropped close on the sides and a little higher on top. He had a square jawline and sharp nose, and every time he turned to smile at his wife, I noticed the dimple on his right cheek. She was pretty, too—a petite woman with a caramel complexion and straight hair, which she wore on this particular Sunday up in a conservative bun. He "Amen-ed" every time the pastor hit his mark.

I was new to this church. I made it my business to

introduce myself to him after the service. When our eyes locked, I knew. He looked at me just a little too long.

Mike worked for a mental-health organization in the Midwest and was a member of a Greek fraternity, a deacon in his church, and well liked. We hit it off instantly. I invited Mike to go with me to a card party, where he had a great time. Afterward we went back to my place, and soon we were making that connection. We didn't get into anything too deep. He was not feeling me like I was feeling him. Instead of becoming sex buddies, we became good friends. He and his wife, who was six weeks pregnant, would hang out with me and my lady friend. Later, when I had my kids for weekend visits, I would take them over to Mike and Sheila's house. Mike and I talked on the phone every day and would share some personal secrets. We became so close that I would let Mike use my apartment to get with his dude. I spent a lot of time out of town, so I gave him a set of keys, and he was free to do whatever in my space. His office was about a block from my place, so it was easy for him and his dude to slip away during lunchtime. His wife loved me and never suspected what either of us was up to. In her mind, if Mike was with me, he was cool because I was cool.

One evening Mike showed up at my house, crying. He was so upset he could barely hold himself up. He told me that he had applied to have his life insurance increased by $250,000. With their baby on the way, Mike wanted to make sure that his family would be properly taken care of. But he had to take a complete physical to qualify. Mike told me he got a call that afternoon from the insurance company telling him he had been declined for the increase.

He said, "J., the only reason they would decline me is if my HIV test came back positive." A lot of times the only way a man finds out he's HIV positive is when he either donates blood or goes for a physical for a life insurance policy, which includes an HIV test. Mike said the doctor's office also called and wanted to talk to him about the results of his physical.

"J., you know I mess around with dudes." He was a bottom (meaning he liked to be penetrated).

"Do you use condoms?" I asked him, knowing the answer, but not knowing what else to say.

"You know I don't use no condoms," he said. "My dude is cool. He's clean. He has a wife, too. And he told me he was just fucking me."

That's a classic line. If you're living on the down low, or DL, and you're lying to your wife or your girlfriend, then there's no reason why you wouldn't lie to every dude you're sleeping with, too.

"Man, what are you going to do?" I asked him.

"What do you think I should do?"

"Bro, tell you what I think. Let's say you contracted it from a woman. Even better, why don't you tell your wife that when you were on a business trip in Las Vegas, you picked up a prostitute, and the condom broke. Ask for forgiveness for that one night of indiscretion. She'll believe that."

"You think they'll believe that, J.?" Mike asked.

"Bro, trust me," I said. "It will work."

The next day Mike went to the doctor, and it was confirmed that he was HIV positive. He told his wife, his family, and his church the story we'd come up with at my house, and they believed him. They forgave him. The church prayed over him. He kept his job. He kept his life. The black community could accept that this brother got the virus from a woman—even a prostitute. They could never accept that he got it from a man.

Mike lost his lover, though. The dude wouldn't even return his phone calls. He cut Mike off and left him to fend for himself, with his wife and kid-to-be. Mike, thank God, is still alive today, and his wife and baby are healthy. His scare and my assistance in covering up the truth were my wake-up call. It was getting too close to home, and

I didn't want to attend another funeral—especially not my own.

Mike's visit was my final straw. Months before, I had had a vision. I was told that my mission was to be honest and to tell my story, but I didn't listen at first. It was a message I didn't understand, nor was it a message I was trying to hear, because I wasn't ready yet to come clean.

At the time, I was a vice president of marketing and sales and sat on the executive board of an African American educational publishing company. I was making six figures and, as part of my package, had use of an expensive house in an upscale Atlanta suburb and a Mercedes-Benz. I had a beautiful apartment and a new Mazda 626 in Columbus, Ohio, and I traveled back and forth between Ohio and Atlanta. I felt I had too much to lose.

Years later, I was still lying even after my wife caught me with another man and divorced me. I never stopped doing what I was doing. I was walking around seeing how many men *and* women I could sleep with. I was caught up with self. It was all about me.

Once I was divorced, I was like a kid in a candy shop. I was going to adult bookstores, churches, anywhere I knew men were—just to pick up brothers. At the same time, I always had a steady girlfriend with whom I was having sex. But things started to change when I got that vision. I started taking a look at who I was, and I didn't like me. In fact, I hated me.

One night I went home and was getting ready to go to sleep, when suddenly I got on my knees and said my prayers. Afterward I got in bed. As I was lying there, my body froze and I couldn't move. My body was in a coma-like state. I was awake and scared. I heard a voice say to me, "You must tell your story."

What?! What was happening to me?

I was fighting to move, but I couldn't. I was sweating and started to panic.

Tell my story? No way!

I eventually came out of this state after what seemed like hours but was probably only a few minutes. Once again as I was lying in bed, the same feeling came over me.

I cannot do this.

I sat on the edge of the bed and started thinking about my daughter, my son, my father, my brother—all the people to whom I would have to expose my life, and I couldn't do it. I couldn't be butt naked before the world. The next day I had a business meeting with a close friend from my church whom I trusted and who knew about my DL life. I told him about the voice I'd heard.

"You know what, Brother King? The pastor has

wanted to hold a men's retreat to discuss why a few of the married sisters in our church are ending up with HIV," he said. And you would be perfect to facilitate this workshop, this men's retreat. The pastor does not want to market it as a homosexual workshop, because he knows the men won't show up. This is your opportunity. If God is speaking to you, this is your calling. Why don't you do this retreat?"

"I can't do that," I said. "I can't go before my church brothers and tell them the truth. I can't do it."

The church didn't have the retreat, and over time more sisters and brothers who I knew were getting HIV. I had been to more funerals that year than I care to remember for members of that church, and friends who attend that church and other churches.

I finally got the message the third time the voice spoke to me. I knew I had to be obedient. I could no longer run. I had decided to move ahead and tell my secrets, along with the secrets of all the black men living double lives and having sex with men *and* women.

Saving lives. It should have been the easiest decision to make. But actually doing it, going out there, was the hardest. I spent two weeks trying to figure out reasons I *shouldn't* do this. I thought about my family. My mother had passed that January, and I knew that if she were still alive, I could never do this. My dad and I were never on the same page about anything, especially my relationships. He was on me shortly after my divorce about having a woman in my life, questioning why my relationships didn't last more than a couple of dates. My younger brother and I were as distant as could be, and we had never had a conversation about anything personal. Ever.

I knew I could deal with their backlash and what they might say about my stepping out. I was sure they would talk about it at my cousin's farm, where the family goes for gatherings and cookouts. I went when my mother was alive but didn't plan to go again. I never felt part of the brotherhood of my male cousins; there was never a connection.

The biggest hurdle I would face would be my ex-wife and my children, especially my children. That is what kept me in a constant psychological tug-of-war. What would my kids say? What would their mother say? How would I face them? How could I explain to them that I needed to tell the world about my life, my secrets, my personal lifestyle? How could I tell them everything that I had hidden from them? What would be the best way to tell them? I prayed, and I asked God for a message, a message that would guide me through this.

In 2001 I decided to resign from my job and had a friend

put together a brochure for me that I called "Secrets of the African American Bisexual Man." I knew "DL" was an undercover word, and health officials wouldn't understand "down low." So I used "bisexual" because that would be a hook to get me in the door. On the cover I put a quotation that read: "Oh, no! Why didn't he tell me?" And inside I gave a brief breakdown of the life of a brother living on the DL.

I wasn't a health expert. I didn't know much about HIV and AIDS or the statistics, but I did know that too many people were dying unnecessarily. I wasn't sure where to start or really where I was going. I just asked to be led. I had been in marketing just about my entire professional career, so I knew how to do this part of it. I sent my brochure to fifty-two health departments throughout the country. Not one responded. I did another mailing. I finally got a call from a director at the Ohio Department of Health, Juliet Dorris-Williams. She said she had received my brochure and wanted to talk with me. I went to the health department and met with her, and her first question was "What is this secret?"

"The secret is that men who look like me, talk like me, and think like me are having sex with men but still love and want to be with their women. And they do not believe they're gay."

"What?!" she said. "Are you willing to say that publicly?"

"I don't know. I'm just stepping out on blind faith. I don't have any credentials. I just know I have a story to tell. I'm a man who leads a double life. I have unprotected sex with men and women. It's only by the grace of God that I'm alive now. Based on my behavior, I should have been dead a long time ago. But I'm willing to share my story with you folks, you professionals who are trying to figure out what's going on."

She schooled me on the numbers—the statistics—and I was chilled to my bones. According to the Centers for Disease Control (CDC), the AIDS rate among black women is three times higher than among Latina women and eighteen times higher than among white women. Today black women make up more than half of all women who have died from AIDS in the United States. African Americans make up 13 percent of the population, yet we now account for nearly 50 percent of all new AIDS cases in the United States. Sixty-eight percent of all new AIDS cases are black women, 75 percent of whom contracted the disease from heterosexual sex.

In the past, the CDC did not separate bisexual and gay behaviors. Both were grouped together, and gay overshadowed bisexual behavior. People saw AIDS still as just a white gay disease. However, the women getting infected were your everyday women, housewives and mothers. Heterosexual sex was being reported as the primary reason for these alarming numbers. Numbers that forced the CDC to take a look at this behavior, and to realize that in the black community, many men did not identify themselves as gay or bisexual, but they were having sex with men.

I put a face and a name to the behavior that was infecting some of our women. It's called the DL—the down low—brothers who have sex with other brothers. They're not in the closet; they're behind the closet. They are so far removed from attaching themselves and what they do to the homosexual lifestyle that these men do not consider themselves gay.

The CDC had not identified why black women were contracting the virus in such high numbers, but I knew one of the reasons. Men who are having unprotected sex with men but *not* labeling themselves gay are also having unprotected sex with women, thus spreading the virus. Women are getting infected by their husbands and boyfriends, who are not telling them that they are also having sex with men. These men are living life on the down low.

In 2000 a CDC study of 8,780 HIV-positive men who said that they were infected by having sex with other men found that 25 percent of African American respondents identified themselves as heterosexual. In contrast, the number of white men who identified themselves as heterosexual while having sex with men was only 6 percent.

The next day I got a call from the Mississippi State Department of Health, which had gotten a call from Ohio about me. They invited me to be their keynote speaker for their World AIDS Day. Craig Thompson, a director at the Mississippi State Department of Health, said he had received my first brochure in the mail. However, during a planning meeting with the program committee, he was urged not to respond.

Thompson said the black women were livid, saying things like "How dare you bring this black man to Mississippi to talk about men who have sex with men!" They thought black men already have too many strikes against them—they are undereducated, so many are in the prison system, and now I wanted to bring this. They threatened to go to the governor's office if Thompson brought me in.

Members of the black gay male community didn't want anything to do with me either. They said they had never heard of me and that the state shouldn't spend its valuable money on somebody who may not be telling the truth. But Thompson said he knew there was something to what I was talking about. Based on his conversations with Juliet Dorris-Williams, he knew that my message and my story could make a difference in his state's HIV-prevention efforts.

"Under all this adversity, Mr. King, would you still be willing to come to Jackson, Mississippi, and share your story?" Thompson asked me. I said yes.

When I got to Mississippi, I was greeted by a whole lot of hostility. Craig Thompson told me that people had written the governor complaining about my being invited to speak. Local ministers urged their congregations to boycott my speech, but despite these efforts the place was packed. Thompson informed me that because of all the controversy, he didn't think it would be wise for me to be the keynote speaker, but asked if I would sit on a workshop panel instead.

The room in which the workshop was held had a capacity of about 50 people, but there were more than 75 people trying to get into the room. Folks lined the walls and stood in the hallway.

It was a bit overwhelming, especially for my first real speaking engagement. There wasn't much structure to the workshop, so I just shared my story about how I was married, how I lied to my wife, how I was having sex with men behind her back, and how I lost my marriage because of this need to have sex with men. I talked about how I didn't like wearing condoms and didn't think much about HIV and AIDS while I was having sex with men. I told them about how women would have sex with me and not even ask me to wear a condom. I broke down the top-and-bottom thing. I told them how I pick up brothers, married brothers, brothers with children and girlfriends, even brothers in that very room (because I knew there was a DL brother or two in the room). I told them how I was a respected member of my community, a member of good standing in my church, and a good father. I also told them I'm not gay.

People were stunned, shocked. Afterward it was a total meltdown, and the line to speak to me was out the door. I met sisters who said they'd lost their husbands to men.

As part of my research—through focus groups, e-mails, workshops, and personal relationships—I have spoken with more than a thousand men from all over the country living on the down low. One is a fifty-eight-year-old minister with three adult children. He is widowed and dates sisters in the church, hoping to find the next first lady. He also has sex with men, and he told me he rarely has protected sex. This brother is educated, mature, and handsome, a great orator, and he's on the DL.

I will share not only my experiences in this book but also the stories of other brothers. Over the last three years, I've met and had discussions with hundreds of men all over this country to find out what compels them to live life on the DL. In order to protect the privacy of the men and women I've spoken with, their names have been changed, along with many of their personal characteristics, including their physical descriptions, professions, and geographical locales.

When you finish this book, I hope you will have a clearer picture of what a DL brother looks like and be open to having more candid discussions about sex with your mate.

2

"BUT I'M NOT GAY!"

I got caught. But many, many men living a double life, living on the DL, never get caught until it's too late. Or if they do get caught, they lie their way out of it or get their wives to forgive them on the promise it will never happen again.

Well, it might happen again. And what's worse, these men—men like I used to be—are selfishly risking the lives of their women and their families. They are having sex with men and bringing home STDs and in some cases the deadly HIV. This behavior is threatening the lives of their wives or girlfriends (and a lot of men have both). These men lie and they cheat. They refuse to let their women go, but they also refuse to give up having sex with men, even when they could lose everything, including their own lives.

How can you explain why so many black heterosexual women in monogamous relationships, in marriages are getting HIV? Many are getting it from their men who are creeping with other brothers, who don't realize they're HIV positive.

Still, a DL friend said to me that he doesn't like the fact that all DL men are being judged and blamed for what is happening. He said that he is not like the others. He protects himself, and most of the time others. He feels that all men should be sexually responsible, but that all men who have sex with both women and men are not promiscuous or sexually irresponsible. All this blame will only keep brothers from disclosing and trusting. A lot of DL and gay men feel, like my friend, that all the blame shouldn't be put on just DL men.

These men may be successful. They may be celebrities. They are husbands, boyfriends, lovers, fathers, and grand-fathers. They attend church and are civic and social leaders. Some have M.D.'s, Ph.D.'s, M.B.A.'s, and law degrees. I have met many police officers, firemen, and even some serving in all branches of the military who live on the down low. They come in all shapes, sizes, and colors. Just walk down any city street or rural small town, and you will see them. You will find them coming out of prison or working in the White House. Some are strong, virile, manly men. They don't fit the stereotypical image of gay men that the media has portrayed. They're not "fags." They're not "punks," and they don't see themselves as *gay*.

To these men gay people are over there—far away from them. Gays march in parades, hang out at gay clubs, go to gay beaches. Gay people may even attend gay churches. They may have the gay flag on their homes and cars.

A gay man knows what he likes in a man. Listening to a gay man talk about his perfect mate is like listening to a woman talk about her perfect man. He can give you in detail what he is looking for in a man. Some gay men will not date or mess with a married man. Others don't care, and it is all about the sex. Open and out gay men are not confused about their sexuality.

Some gay men are in the closet. They are still gay. They just can't admit it publicly, because of family, religion, and/or job. They may be in a fraternity and feel that their frat brothers will not be able to deal with them if it is common knowledge that they are gay. I've heard some say, "My mother would die; it would kill her if she found out." Or maybe they work for a law firm and feel that they won't be taken seriously or get that promotion if everyone knows they are gay. But they are gay. They have a community that is aware of this fact and provides them with a comfortable environment in which to "let their hair down." Perhaps outside their family and job they have places where they can be open about their lifestyle. Maybe when he's on vacation, the closeted gay man finds out where the gay clubs or cruising parks are, and when he's out of town, he can be himself. These brothers accept their gayness, but their love and respect for their family or fear may force them to stay in the closet. Even when they admit to close family and friends that they have same-sex feelings, they will go ahead with the front, to save face or name or to make others happy. But they don't enjoy sex with women, because they are *gay*.

Then there are bisexual men—they want it all. A bisexual man may tell his girlfriend or wife, "Look, baby, I like a little spice in my life," or "I am open. I don't have any hang-ups with sex. Sex is sex." He may suggest that a third party join them—man or woman.

Then there are men like I used to be—DL men. They are so undercover, so in denial, so "on the low" that they are *behind* the closet. A new term has been created by the HIV-prevention industry to describe the DL man: "non-ID MSM," or non-identified men who sleep with men. These brothers don't even want to be called DL. They will not openly admit their desires for men. Even if caught in bed with another man, a DL man will deny that anything remotely homosexual is going on. He will blame it on drugs, liquor, the lack of sex from his woman, depression, his weakness, or the need for attention—anything but being a homosexual. "Denial" is the operative word.

Then there are straight men (a.k.a. heterosexuals), who I believe are in the majority. A straight man would never look twice at another man.

But a DL man fronts with women. He's the one you see at the clubs, buying women drinks, dancing with the sisters, and getting them all worked up. He may not even hook up with a brother (that night) in that environment unless he makes eye contact with one and they exchange signals. For the most part, the DL man is indistinguishable from every other man in the crowd. And that's the way he likes it.

DL men cannot and will not be associated with anything that would raise any questions about his sexuality. They will not say they are gay, because those three little letters evoke so much fear. Those three letters have them afraid of being ostracized by their community, by their church, by their family. If they tell the truth and say they're gay or bisexual, they will be called a "fag." That's the worst word you can call a black man. When a man is called a fag, it hurts. It basically strips away your manhood.

You're saying I'm less than a man. You're saying I'm soft, that I want to be a woman or that I act like a woman.

When you think of gay, you think of RuPaul or '70s singer Sylvester or Blaine and Antoine, the very feminine critics in "Men on Film" from *In Living Color. That's* gay. You can be a big, buffed pro-football player or a critically acclaimed actor, but if you tell anyone that you sleep with men, all your accomplishments go out the window. You become the gay football player or the gay actor. You can be a popular basketball all-star player, but once you show even a hint of liking men sexually, you become the gay basketball player.

There have been several white movie stars, athletes, politicians, and business leaders who have come out, and continue to do their job without the backlash. It's a helluva lot easier for white folks to accept homosexuality, because they have their "out" Elton Johns and Ellens, their *Queer as Folk* and *Will and Grace.* They're not tripping. Could a famous, popular black athlete ever come out like the Olympic diver Greg Louganis did and get the same treatment? I don't think so.

When I was growing up in Springfield, Ohio, every gay man, as I recall, was sad. Brother Jones, who played the piano at churches around the city, was a flamboyant older man, who even in my youth was weird to me. Two or three boys in my school were gay. And nobody liked them. No one picked them to be a part of any sports teams. No one wanted to be in the locker room or in the showers with them. They were constantly beaten up and called "fag." Even today, young men who have this sexual confusion hear and see those young men and the ways they're constantly ostracized, and it affects them deeply.

If you're gay, people don't want to leave their sons around you, because they're afraid you might molest them. People think gay men want sex all the time, wherever they can get it. People look at you like you have AIDS.

If I admit I'm gay, my son's friends will look at him differently. If I'm gay or bisexual, every time they talk about some gay thing on television, some gay bashing, or some gay issue, you'll think about me. I don't want that. If I say I'm gay, every time I'm in your presence and a brother comes up to us, you'll make those little comments, "Isn't *he* cute?" Or something stupid like "I saw you looking at his ass." You'll throw me into that whole culture, and I'm not going out like that. I'm not going to let you do that to me.

To a lot of men, to admit being gay is to ask for a life of hell and abuse. Who wants that? They would rather stay on the DL.

To this day, even though I'm honest with those in my life about my sexual habits, I will not be labeled gay. If I admit that, then I'm giving up and buying into a lifestyle and a label that I do not believe define me. People want me to say I am gay. That would make them feel better, feel more comfortable with me. If I would just say I am gay, then they could deal with me. Put me over there with "them" and return to their lives. I become okay as a gay man, because gay men don't have sex with women. But that's not who I am. I do have sex with women.

When I am asked today about my sexual orientation, or what am I now that I am no longer on the DL, I tell them that I am a man who formally lived a DL lifestyle, secretly having sex with men while maintaining relationships with women. I lived under the shadow of lies, being deceitful and using women to cover up my bisexual behavior. For a long while, I never gave any thought to the pain that I caused others whom I loved or cared about. Neither the women I became involved with nor my family came before my need to fulfill my sexual desire for men. Ultimately, it was my strong love and respect for women that caused me to come clean. When I looked at my adult daughter, my nieces, cousins, and many women friends, I knew that I could no longer allow them to remain victims of this behavior. Coming clean would be a major step, but I had to do it.

I don't consider myself gay, and how I define my sexual identity is my choice. I respect the identity choices that others make. I know who I am and I have made peace with myself. I no longer have to hide or lie about who I am. And for this, I am grateful to God. I want to be a positive example for men who are living in the turmoil of a double life. I want them to know that life is more peaceful and guilt-free when we are in integrity with women and honor their right to choose whether or not they want to share their body, soul, and love with a man who isn't exclusively heterosexual. As I look back on my journey, I realize that I am not the man who started out as a spokesperson for the DL community. I am no longer proud of that part of my life.

A DL man doesn't like gay behavior. He will not be caught around anyone or anything that even looks gay. He's the first one to stand up in church and shout, "Get the homosexuals out of here!" He's the first one to call someone a "faggot." He's the one who says, "My son better not ever be a fag. I will beat him straight!" He is verbal about his dislike of gays and homosexuals. Publicly he is disgusted by the idea that two men would have sex with each other.

Women involved with DL men are being infected with HIV because these men do not believe in wearing condoms and they don't know their HIV status. Condoms take away from the very thing they are seeking—the thrill of spontaneity. Condoms take away that feeling when having man-to-man sex. To put on a condom is to think about what you're doing. It stops it from being a thoughtless, lustful act that they have no control over. If you wear a condom, it couldn't be the liquor that made you have sex with a man.

And even if they thought to wear one with their ladies, how in the world could they explain that? His wife or steady girlfriend thinks they have a monogamous relationship. How does he then slip on a condom without a lot of explaining?

But for the most part, a man on the DL isn't even thinking about all that. He's not thinking about a condom or diseases. DL men look at themselves as invincible, strong black men. They ain't catching that "gay disease." When you talk about HIV and AIDS to them, you're talking about those limp-wristed people. "They aren't talking about me," they're convinced.

When a DL man is out having sex with men, he's not debating whether or not he's gay or bisexual. He has only one thing on his mind: Let me do this and get home to my woman before she wakes up, gets off work, comes home, or starts missing me.

At the 2002 International AIDS Conference held in Barcelona, Spain, one of the panels was titled "Confronting Challenges of Prevention Outreach to Non-Identified MSM of Color." Translation: How do we reach these men of color (these black men) who do not identify themselves as gay yet have sex with men? That is the biggest challenge right now for HIV-prevention workers, because the heterosexual community—mostly black women—is becoming the fastest-growing demographic to contract HIV.

According to a recent study conducted by the Michigan Department of Community Health and the Centers for Disease Control, black and Hispanic women are getting HIV at a higher rate than the rest of the population, because many of them don't realize their male lovers are having sex with men. It's this lack of awareness that causes women to leave themselves open to infection by having unprotected sex with their men.

When I was still in my DL behavior, knowing my HIV status was not a consideration. I didn't want to know. I just prayed that I was clean. I reasoned that if I was infected, I'd wait until I got sick or dropped dead. I didn't talk to anyone about having an HIV/AIDS test, and what that could mean for saving my life. I became my own worst enemy. I'd wait until later, or I'd wait until there were some signs. I wasn't losing weight; I felt good, looked well, and that was all that mattered to me. To know that I had HIV would be a living hell, and I didn't want to know. So the hell with taking a test. I know that a lot of men who have put themselves at risk have had this same conversation with themselves. Getting tested is not a conversation that comes up at parties, at the club, church, or when men are together at the gym. There are billboards, signs on buses and the train, and ads on TV, but men at risk block out those messages.

I didn't want to think about my behavior or the risk. I didn't want to know. I just wanted to forget about it, until the next time. This rotating door is what many DL men go through every day, even when they know what the test results would be. Some sisters end up being the "lab rat," and when they get infected their men know that they must be as well. What a sacrifice.

3.

WAS MY MARRIAGE A LIE?

I walked to the door of my house as I had done
every day since we bought the beautiful fixer-
upper in one of the most prestigious black neigh-
borhoods in our town. I was feeling really good as I put
the key in the door, looking forward to enjoying a quiet
evening with my wife and our two children. The key, however, wasn't working. I tried it several times, and it
wouldn't budge. Finally I had to ring the doorbell. My
brother-in-law, my wife's youngest brother, opened it
hard.

"You better get your faggot ass out of here before I
f—— you up!" he yelled.

What?!

My heart started beating fast, and I broke out into an instant sweat as I stood on the front porch of my own house with my brother-in-law inches from my face. One of my best friends, who lived across the street, had come out of his house to get rid of the trash. He waved and yelled out, "What's up, man!" But I didn't pay him any attention. I was trying to figure out what was going on at *my* house. I then started to think about the lady who lived next door. She was a member of the church my mother attended. Miss Odell was like the character Pearl from the 1980s situation comedy *227*, the one who would hang out the window and get in everybody's business. My wife and I would laugh about how she probably looked through her bedroom window at us each night, checking our every move. So I just knew she caught the showdown between my brother-in-law and me and was probably on the phone calling my mother, or other folks in the church, at that very moment.

My brother-in-law continued to block my path, but I looked around him into the kitchen, where I saw my sisters-in-law huddled around my wife, who was crying. John continued to block me out, and I was getting angrier and angrier. I never liked him anyway. He was my least favorite of my five brothers-in-law. Now he was standing in my doorway, controlling my house, and that pissed me off more than anything—more than having to leave, which is what I ended up doing.

My mind was racing during the five-minute drive to my parents' house (where else was I going to go?). I was trying to retrace my day. What had happened between leaving that morning for work, with a kiss from my wife and kids, and coming home that evening that so dramatically altered my life?

Of course, I knew exactly what I had done that day. But how in the world did Brenda find out? How could she possibly know?

Instead of going to my class, as I had told my wife I was doing every afternoon, I went to Melvin Gregory's house. Melvin was an older man I met in church who took me under his wing. When Brenda and I moved back to our hometown after being overseas and in Texas, he seemed to seek me out. He asked me to help him with a men's mentoring program he was starting at the church. I was happy to do it. I never had a tight relationship with my dad— who was an excellent provider but didn't really have much conversation or emotional support for me—so meeting Brother Gregory gave me an opportunity to hang out with an older father-figure type and perhaps get some paternal love. I was also flattered that he wanted *me* to help him on his mentoring project.

One Sunday after church I rode to his house on my bi-
cycle to discuss the men's ministry. We lived in a small
town—everything seemed practically within walking distance. Why waste the gas, I thought, and the bike was also
a good way for me to get some exercise. I parked my bike
in his backyard and went inside, and he offered me a
drink. It was a hot summer day, and I expected water or
lemonade. Instead, Melvin pulled out a bottle of E&J, a
cheap brandy. We talked for a while, and before I knew it,
we had finished half the bottle. We talked a little about
the church's mentoring program, but by the way Melvin
was looking at me, I could tell he might have another kind
of mentoring in mind.

"Do you like videos?" he asked me.

I told him I did.

"Why don't you come upstairs," he said. "There are
some videos I want to show you."

His videos were of men having sex. At this point I am
E&J'd out and feeling it. I was just going with the flow. I
was a little shocked, but I was also getting very turned
on. I was high on his bed, watching a video of men having
sex. I was starting to get aroused, and before I even noticed, Melvin had slipped beside me and started lightly
kissing my neck and making me even more aroused. I did
not resist. He took it further and began to undress me. I

still did not resist. As he started kissing my chest and rubbing my erection, he took off his clothes, and we began to have sex. No words were exchanged.

Afterward I slept off my high—both highs—and left. Melvin had awakened something in me that I thought would never take bloom. As long as I could remember, I have had some attraction to men, but I never acted on it before this day. But after that day I had a desire to see Melvin every chance I could. I was open, hooked. It was like a drug that I could not get enough of. The more he gave me, the more I wanted. Melvin was satisfying my sexual desire, touching me in ways I had never been touched before and anticipating what I wanted even before I knew myself. It was like being with a mind-blowing mind reader. Can you imagine having someone fulfill sexual desires you didn't even know you had?

Melvin was perfect for me. He lived nearby, my wife liked him, he was respected in the community, he lived alone, and he had a high sex drive. I liked the way Melvin made me feel. He was an elegant man. He was a cool older brother who loved Billie Holiday and Ella Fitzgerald. His home had a spiral staircase and a fireplace. Going to his house was what I lived for. There were liquor, music, and a strong desire for my body.

Being with him was an escape to a world I didn't think

existed. Even though things were perfect at home, being with Melvin completed everything. I had a great job and family, and now I had someone I could let my guard down with and totally be myself. I could allow those desires and feelings that I had for so long tried to bury and kill come out and breathe. I knew those feelings of wanting to be with another brother were not dead; they were just asleep. They were not gone but on vacation. They were simply locked away. Melvin found the key, and I allowed him to unlock that door.

Looking back, I don't know if I would ever have approached him. But he must have seen something in my eyes. He must have noticed the way I looked at him. I know he felt when we were watching videos that it would be okay for him to continue. I'm sure my body was telling him to make his move. Melvin was a pro. He had his Ph.D. in DL behavior. Compared with him, I was still in grade school. He was divorced and had a string of lady friends on the side, but he had years of experience in the DL life. He knew to take his time with me. No, he didn't waste any time making the initial move, but when he actually got down to business, Melvin was slow and steady. I just followed his lead.

We didn't just have sex. Melvin was turning out to be a good friend. He listened to me. I was able to talk with him about things, and he seemed to have all the answers, and he knew when to be quiet. He knew I was confused about my sexual desires, but he never once talked about my family, and we never discussed what we were doing. We did what we did sexually with few words. Not one time did we talk about what we were doing as being gay or homosexual. In fact, we never even talked about safe or safer sex. We never used protection. Never. He schooled me in the fine art of having sex with a man, but he never taught me how to be safe or how to be on the DL and not get caught.

Several months into my involvement with Melvin, I started getting really comfortable and sloppy and cocky. It was easy to be cocky when things were going so perfectly in my world. I had the perfect wife, who was also a perfect mother. She didn't miss a beat in supporting me emotionally and was there for me in every way a woman can be.

The deeper I got with Melvin, the more I started to neglect Brenda. I became distant. Our sex life was different—strained. She wondered why I wasn't as affectionate as I used to be and why I wasn't making love to her as frequently. When I told her I was stressed with work and school and still adjusting to civilian life in my hometown, she understood. She didn't pressure me. When she wondered why I spent so much time away from home, I explained that being back in town, I had so many people to catch up with—my folks, my friends from high school. And she understood. She knew that I was in school and that I worked hard. I took her kindness and understanding as an opportunity to do whatever I wanted. That was one of many mistakes I made. The first one was sleeping with Melvin.

In the beginning I would never park my car in his driveway or anywhere near his house, because his driveway and house were too open and exposed. I would park down the street and walk to his place or ride my bike and keep it in the back. But after I got caught up in Melvin's world and my own arrogance, I stopped thinking about who might ride by and see my car. I started parking right in front of his door (a big no-no).

That's where my car was the day Brenda caught me. My car was there all afternoon. It was also there all afternoon the day before, when one of Brenda's friends spotted it—I later found out—and called her. I was supposed to be in class both days. When I got home the evening of the day Brenda's friend saw my car at Melvin's, Brenda asked me how class was.

"Baby, it was a tough day," I told her. "The professor was on me all class."

I was busted in a lie. But Brenda never let on that she knew I was lying. Instead, she went into detective mode. She went through my wallet that night and found a picture of Melvin. I had stupidly begged him for a photo (another big no-no). She was now suspicious enough to see for herself where I was actually going every afternoon instead of class.

The next day I went to Melvin's, as I had been doing for months. I had long since dropped my class. Sometime during my visit to Melvin's, Brenda drove over. I was boldly parked in the driveway, because I had not planned on staying long—at least that's what I'd told myself. I walked up the steps and called to Melvin as I opened his front door. In our small town it was not unusual for people to leave their doors unlocked. After I went in, I didn't even think about locking the door. I went up to the bedroom, which faced the stairs. Before I reached the top, I could see Melvin lying naked across the queen-size bed, waiting for me.

He smelled good, and he was ready to get into a little something-something. There was no liquor this day but plenty of foreplay—Melvin's specialty. I didn't think it was possible for a person to be so gentle and smooth yet so intense and strong. Just as strong was the music blaring from the sound system, a wild jazz beat that seemed to keep time with what we were doing in the room. It was almost primal. I was in another world. Lost.

We were both so caught up in what we were doing that neither one of us noticed that someone had come in the front door. Neither one of us heard the footsteps on the stairs leading to the bedroom, nor did we hear those same footsteps rush back out. That day we had an unexpected audience that would cost me my marriage and the life I dearly loved.

Brenda had to see for herself what her friend had reported. She saw my car—my raggedy gold Cutlass—in front of Melvin's house. She came to the front door. Maybe she knocked. The music was so loud it could be heard from the street, and it would have been impossible to hear a knock. She knew I was inside, so maybe she tried the knob and found the front door open. She must have followed the sound of the music, which led her upstairs. With the music and the mood going, Brenda probably got an eyeful—more than enough evidence, more than enough to know that Melvin and I weren't just talking about a mentoring program. When she got home, she called her sisters and her brothers, and they all came to her rescue.

While I was at Melvin's thinking that all was well at home, my wife was pulling in her family to protect her from me, her husband—this man who she had just found out was a stranger to her, this person whom she had been married to for seven years, her first lover, her high-school sweetheart, her prom date, the first man whom her father allowed her to be in a serious relationship with, the father of her children, the man she trusted with her life, the man who promised to grow old with her. Now all that was a lie. Her marriage was a lie, and she had been living all those years with a stranger.

As I said, after the showdown with John I got in my car and headed to my parents' house. I thought about going back to Melvin's but knew that would not be a smart move. In fact, I would never go to Melvin's again. So Mom's it was. I had nobody else to talk to, to get advice from, no place to hide out until this "thing" blew over. I really thought it would blow over. In my twisted mind I was still the man Brenda loved. And while I wasn't perfect, I thought she would take me back. Whatever was going on, it couldn't stamp out our love. I decided to go to my parents' until she came to her senses. I would go there and act like nothing was wrong.

As I got closer to the house I grew up in, tears started flowing. I cried so hard I wasn't sure I would ever stop. Deep inside I knew that I had messed up and that it was serious. When I pulled up in front of my parents' house, I noticed they were not sitting on the front porch, as they did every evening before they went to bed. I wiped my eyes and tried to pull myself together before I went into the house. I was an emotional wreck. I had always been emotional, especially when I talked to my mom about issues that bothered me. She would always baby me and look at me with eyes that saw straight through me with understanding. She had that way about her, and she always knew how I was really feeling.

When I got inside the house, I discovered that my parents were upstairs in their respective bedrooms. My mom and dad hadn't slept in the same room for years. My dad had taken over the room once shared by my brother and me, while my mom had the master bedroom across the hall. When I got to the top of the stairs, I saw my dad sitting on his bed with his head in his hands. He had been crying and was shaking his head back and forth, saying something under his breath that I couldn't quite make out.

I headed straight for my mother's room. She was lying on her bed, crying. She had just gotten off the phone with Brenda, who told her, "Our marriage was a lie!" She told my mother she was filing for divorce and wanted custody of the kids. Divorce? That was not even in my parents' vocabulary. They were confused, but they knew that my life was about to change and they were afraid.

For my father it was about the reputation of the family and *his* reputation in the church.

"You have embarrassed the family," he said to me. "Why did you do this? People are going to talk about us. How am I going to face my church? Why did you do this?!"

He didn't want to hear anything from me. As far as he was concerned, I had ruined the family name. In a small town news travels fast, especially news like "Jimmy King is a fag!" That would be on the front page: "The perfect King family had a black mark. Yeah, that son Deacon and Mrs. King bragged so much about, who never got in trouble, who had served his country, got married and was raising a beautiful family, bought a house, and was now going back to school, that son is a fag. The one who could do no wrong has fallen from grace." That's the way the story would go.

I sat on the edge of my mom's bed, laid my head on her chest, and started crying again. This time the cry came from another place. It was a cry I can't explain. I wasn't crying because I had done this thing and ruined my family. I was crying because I had gotten caught. As each tear fell,

I was plotting how I would make it all right and undo the damage. I was going to get out of this and get things back to normal. Even in the middle of this emotional roller coaster, my spirit was not defeated. I was going to return to my home and family.

It was all about me. I was not worried about my children; they were young, and this would not impact them yet, I thought. I was in the "now" mode. I had to regroup and do so quickly.

I moved in with my parents, one of the hardest things to do. I had not lived with them since high school, and I had grown accustomed to having my freedom. Now I was back in my old room—moving my dad back in with my mother—and under constant watch. I went into a deep depression. I stopped eating and couldn't sleep. My mother was concerned about my health—both physical and mental.

I missed my children. I missed my wife. I also missed my life. Brenda wouldn't let me talk to my kids, let alone talk to her. When I called, one of her sisters would always answer the phone. If Brenda ever did pick up and heard it was me, there was no conversation. She would say, "I want to end this marriage!" and hang up.

I used to drive by my house to try to get a glimpse of my children or Brenda. I never saw them. Brenda had sent the children to stay with one of her sisters for "safe keeping." This was hurting not only me but also my parents, who did nothing to deserve being locked out of their grandchildren's lives. Before this, my mother talked to and saw her grandchildren every day. My children spent more time with my parents than they did with Brenda and me. I could see the hurt on my mother's face at not being able to see her babies. I had to do something to get my family back together.

I decided I would woo Brenda, as I did when we first started dating. I would be more in touch with her feelings and sensitive to everything she was going through. I stopped thinking about me. And I definitely wasn't thinking about Melvin. All those feelings and desires were dead. I even refused to drive down the street where he lived, and I stopped going to the church I had attended with my wife. I just sat in my room thinking about what I had done to myself and to my family.

After several weeks Brenda began to soften a bit. She started talking to me but would always end our conversations with the same request to dissolve the marriage. She wanted me to admit that I was unfaithful and that the marriage was a seven-year lie. She told me that if I did that, she would not expose me further. I refused to accept her offer. I didn't want to lose her. I planned on fighting for my marriage. I was determined that she would take me back. And during those weeks apart, after my grieving ended, I had somehow convinced myself that Brenda was wrong for trying to tear up our marriage. How could she do this to our children? I was not going away without a fight.

Brenda stood firm, though, and refused to bend. My mother tried to talk to her. That didn't work. We went to our pastor for guidance, and he told her to stand by her man. That didn't work. I sent her a dozen roses. That didn't work. When we were together, I tried to make love to her. That definitely didn't work. She was through with me. And she had the complete support of her family to keep her strong. Because she was the baby of a large family, every one of her siblings rallied around to protect her, like a solid wall to keep me from her. The tension between my family and her family was so thick I thought it might turn into an all-out family feud.

Even with the rumors about what I did, I managed to convince my family that Brenda's family was standing in the way of our reconciling. They were the ones keeping us from the children. They were the ones hurting us. Brenda's family had the upper hand—they had my children, my house, my possessions.

Finally, three months after the "incident," divorce papers were served to me. I had to face the reality. We were not getting back together. I was only twenty-seven years old, and I was going to be the first person in my family to get a divorce. It was a dark time in my life and the life of my family. During this same period I got laid off from my job and was also on the brink of losing the house. Brenda wanted to keep it, but she could not afford to pay the mortgage. I was not working and couldn't afford the payments and the temporary child support I was ordered to pay. I still had not had any time with my children, which was killing me. Brenda felt that I was not man enough to be a father to my children and that they needed a "real" man to be there for them. She told me they needed her brothers, not me.

We ended up losing the house, the dream house, the house that everybody was so proud of, the house that set us apart from all our high-school friends. That house was the main gathering place for both of our families. Now I would never set foot in it again. Brenda's brothers dropped off my personal possessions at my parents' house.

The divorce took about six months to finalize. During that time I moved out of my parents' house, started dating other women, and discovered Columbus, Ohio's capital and largest city. It was about an hour from my hometown, and there I discovered a new world. Brothers there could meet my sexual need for men, and I could do what I wanted away from my family, my ex-wife, and anybody else who might know me. I had found a new networking opportunity that helped me develop my DL skills even more.

Brenda made the right choice by not taking me back. It was only a matter of time before I was back on the prowl, exploring my sexual desire for men.

4

SHE CAN'T COMPETE WITH HIM

"I'm going to give it to him the way he wants it. I'm going to give him something he'll never forget."

I hear women say this all the time. They feel that if they do their job properly in the bedroom, their man will not have a reason to stray. However, if your man sleeps with men, there is nothing sexually you can do that will make him stop. You can't perform oral sex on your man, or allow him to hit it from the back, or anything else you may think of that will "rock his world." Nothing will make a brother who likes to have sex with other brothers stop. I know that sounds harsh, but it's true. If a man enjoys sex with a man, there's not a woman alive who can compete with that desire, because, it's simple, *she's not a man*.

When a man cheats on his woman with a man, it's often all about sex. The sex is different, and a woman can't duplicate it. That's where many women go wrong. They think there is something *they* can do. Or, worse, they think it's *their* fault that their man is sleeping with a man.

I placed an ad on a Web site calling for men living on the DL to come together—under complete confidentiality—and discuss their lives and why they cheat on their women and sleep with men. Men will lie and say it's the woman's fault. Some brothers complained about their ladies being boring in bed or getting fat. They complained about women not allowing them to go in really deeply when they had sex or about the kids waking up in the middle of the night. They said they were tired of their women's complaining about the bills.

"Man, I just go over to my boy's house, smoke a blunt, get my dick sucked, get my shit off, and I don't have to hear none of that," one guy said. "Then I can go home and deal with her."

I don't believe the reasons these men provided. In my opinion their responses reflect the rationalizing personality of men living on the DL. They do not readily accept responsibility for their actions. They're also searching for motivations and excuses for living this double life. These men's ladies—even with all their issues—don't have anything to do with the need to have sex with other men. I know quite a few DL brothers (including the old me, before I came clean and started being honest with the people in my life) who have tried to convince a woman that it is her fault. These men will talk her into believing that she actually had something to do with their fooling around with men.

I recently had a conversation with a brother who had been married for seven years. When I asked him why he has unprotected sex with a man, he replied, "I trust this man. My wife has been getting on my nerves." He said that when he's with men, it's stress-free. No expectations. No lovemaking. Just sex.

His was a typical cop-out. She didn't drive him to do what he was doing.

"Is she making you put your life at risk? Is she making you put her life at risk?" I asked. He just sat there and looked straight ahead. He didn't have an answer. He was satisfied in deflecting the guilt and blame away from himself.

I did the same thing to my wife. I tried to make her think she was crazy when she caught me. I tried to make all our friends think she was overreacting. "I am a good father and husband. I take care of everything, and she wants to put me through this?!" I would complain. I completely turned the whole thing around to avoid taking responsibility. The bottom line is that I slept with men because that's what I liked—the same as all my down-low brothers.

There is something indescribable about being with a man. A man knows what he likes, so sex with some men is like sex with a mind reader, someone who knows exactly how you like it. I've had brothers perform oral sex on me so well I almost passed out. For some men it's better than anal sex. In the MSM world, oral sex is often preferred because it's safer than unprotected anal sex.

Sex between men is about more than sex; it's also about power. Something about a man's penis says dominance. The penis represents power and control. Some little, dainty-looking guy who is five feet five, weighing a buck twenty-five, can be packing a nine-inch penis. That's power. And it's not even just about the size—although men seem constantly to brag about and focus on the size of their penises.

Whatever the size of a man's penis, it is clear that's where the power is. You may have a really masculine man who sleeps with another man because he wants to be dominated—something he can never be as head of his household. Maybe he wants to be held by a man to feel a certain security in his physical strength that his woman cannot provide. For other men, like me, it's about total domination, raw and rough.

I've heard women say, "I'm going to be his best friend," or "I'm going to be interested in sports," or "I'm going to support his dream." Those things may make your marriage better, but none of them will stop your man—who enjoys sex with men—from having sex with a man. A woman who thinks she will do all these things *for* her man in hopes that he will give her the attention he is showing his boys is wasting her time.

I met Gary during the course of my research. He told me about his experiences living on the DL. He was so deep in this lifestyle, he said, that when he announced he was finally going to get married, all his friends—who were also on the DL—got nervous. He had already called the wedding off three times. He said there were rumors that the real reason he was calling off the wedding was that he was gay. His bride-to-be, Ursula, had heard all the rumors but refused to believe them, or maybe she didn't care. She was getting married.

At the wedding Gary stood proud with his groomsmen, who were all involved the night before in what Gary described as one of the wildest bachelor parties he had ever been to.

On her wedding day Ursula stood with her bridesmaids,

girlfriends from the church and her many social clubs. She was the envy of the other women. She had something that most wanted—a successful, hardworking black man, a true man, a man who loved and cared for her. Gary was not in prison, on drugs, or gay (he couldn't be if he was standing up there marrying her, right?). Ursula had a man who even loved God.

When the pastor pronounced them man and wife, you could hear a pin drop in the church, Gary said. Once they were married, though, things changed. Gary could no longer come and go as he pleased. Ursula became overprotective and insecure about his friends hanging around all the time. At first Gary said he was okay with this. He felt it was time to move away from his DL friends and settle down and have a family. To his credit, he did try to stop. He tried to suppress his desire to be with men. He really did love Ursula. He wanted to make it work. But like every other man I know who lives on the DL, he eventually came back. And when Gary returned to that life, he said, he did so hungrier than ever.

What's really scary about this thing, at least for me, is that the desire to be with other men has such a strong pull that it feels like you can't resist it. It's like something overtakes you. It's insanity. I discussed this with a minis-

ter friend, who describes the lust, the drive as akin to being possessed.

"J., think about this," he said. "When two men are in
the middle of having sex, it's as if their bodies, their spir-
its are taken over. Think about it. When you have sex
with a brother, doesn't your body go through changes and
movements—movements you could never make ordin-
arily? Your face goes through these ugly changes; your
voice even changes. For those five minutes or those
twenty minutes you are not yourself. It's like a demonic
spirit has come into both of you, and that passion is not
who you are."

I shared this with other brothers and asked them if
they ever felt like they were having an out-of-body experience while having sex with a man. Every last one of
them said yes. One person told me, "I never drink, but
when I think about having sex with a man, I need a drink.
I become a different person."

When I get with a brother and I'm feeling it, I'm not
the same person. I know brothers who say they cuss when
they're with other men and they never cuss in their everyday life. You're saying and doing things you could never
imagine yourself saying and doing. And when you're
through, you roll over or get up, and nine out of ten times

you say, "Yo, dude, I gotta go!" You're thinking to yourself, "What did I just do?!"

I tried on many occasions to stop these strong feelings. Every time I looked at my wife and children or women who loved me, and all we had, I thought, "What am I doing?!" "How could I put all of this at risk by pursuing these desires?!" I wasn't thinking about being with brothers at that moment, but as soon as I got in the presence of a man whom I was feeling and who was feeling me, the desire came rushing back, and the women in my life and my children were not at all on my mind.

I've asked all the men I've spoken with throughout the country the following question: If a pill were invented that would make them totally stop this behavior, that would completely erase any and all desire for men, would they take it? Every single one of them said emphatically yes.

Not one brother I talked with said he loves living this way. No one said he loves leading a double life, putting his life and job at risk. I have never heard anyone say, "I love being blackballed," or "I love always being on the prowl, looking for trouble," or "I love getting herpes and having to explain to my wife the blisters on my penis." No one loves having to sneak away to another county to a clinic to get a shot for gonorrhea he contracted from unprotected sex with a man.

Many men go home and sleep with their wives after having sex with a brother because, they say, they feel guilty. They tell me that sometimes they feel so dirty and so guilty when they return home that they feel like they have to get clean by being intimate with their girlfriends or wives. They intensify the lovemaking to compensate for what they did an hour earlier.

When you're in this down-low lifestyle, you are constantly protecting your image. DL brothers have a macho, "ultra-male" image that borders on homophobia. When I was on the DL, I had to be careful with the kind of men I was seen with in public; they could not be remotely flamboyant or "readable," easily detected as being gay. I had to watch my language and try hard not to slip into the kind of verbiage I used when hanging out with my DL friends. I was careful about how I dressed. And when I had lady friends over, I had to make sure that anything that would connect me to that lifestyle was well hidden.

Living on the down low is like living in a fantasy world. As a result of the state of denial, one must constantly reinforce this behavior. In fact, it took me more than twenty years to get real. It took me almost twenty years to apologize to my wife for my deception. Before I started writing this book, I was asked if I had ever apologized to my wife. Before that time I couldn't do it, because it would be admitting that I had done something wrong and that she had been right about everything she had said about me.

I spent a great many of those twenty years blaming her, running and hiding from the truth. I told everyone that *she* was the one who ruined our perfect marriage and our perfect life. I loved her, and she wouldn't take me back. I had promised I would be more attentive to her needs and do anything, and she wouldn't hear it. She wouldn't take me back. She took my children from me. I was telling people that she wasn't there for me, that she wasn't fulfilling my needs. But that was a lie. I would have done anything to take the heat off myself. The truth is it was all my fault. I messed up. My wife, as fine and as pretty and as perfect as she was, was not enough to make me stop having sex with men.

Years after our marriage was dismantled, I got a call from my ex-wife out of the blue. She told me she had seen Melvin in church and that they had spoken with each other for the first time in several years.

"Jimmy, all these years I didn't like him, didn't want to speak to him; I avoided him," Brenda said. "But two

Saturdays ago we caught eyes, and after the service we found each other among the congregation and stood in the middle of the church and hugged and cried.

"I told him, 'I forgive you,' and he told me, 'I'm sorry,' and I could see that he truly was sorry. Jimmy, it felt so good to let all those years and all that pain go."

I responded by saying, "Uh, I got to go, baby. I'll talk to you later." And I hung up. I couldn't handle it. I wasn't ready to face my actions. It was a special moment that she wanted to share with me, and I couldn't handle it. I didn't want to hear it. I sat at my desk motionless for about half an hour.

I was afraid to utter those words, "I'm sorry that I lied to you." I was afraid to admit that the failed marriage was my fault. I was afraid to admit that I had sexual tendencies or behavior that might be *g-a-y*. In my mind, to apologize would be to acknowledge that our marriage was a lie. I still needed to think that Brenda could possibly see me as the perfect man I envisioned being and tried to present to the world.

I am not perfect, and Brenda of all people on earth knows this. If she could forgive Melvin, I knew she could forgive me. To this day, when I'm in a room alone with my ex-wife, I get uncomfortable—even though she's been to my house and she has a new husband. I love her as much today as the day we were married. She says she prays for me. She tells me all the time that she loves me as a child of God and doesn't have hate for me. She says that it's very important that I be honest with everyone in my life. She comes to my defense now when people attack me. She tells her family that she supports me because I am the father of her children, that I was her first love and her first male best friend.

It took her a long time to come to terms with what I had done to our lives. She was so torn emotionally by what I did to her. Brenda told me that for years she could not trust men. Before she remarried, every time her boyfriend left the house, she thought, "Is this going to happen to me again?"

She told me she forgives me and loves me. She said, "You always love the first man you've ever been with. You're a good father to your kids. They love you, and they respect you. What you're doing now, coming clean, will help a lot of women."

I have admitted the truth. The truth is that I am a man who likes having sex with men . . . and women. I have girlfriends with whom I am very upfront. And while being with them will not stop me from sleeping with men, I need them in my life. I give them the choice. I don't make this decision for them. I don't try and play God.

5

I LOVE THE LADIES, TOO

I was invited to be a keynote presenter at Delta Sigma Theta sorority's 2001 Eastern Regional Conference in Baltimore. On the day I was scheduled to speak, I arrived at the hotel early. There was plenty of time to check out the hotel *and* the ladies. I came to the convention ready, in prowl mode. My purpose was to see how many numbers I could get.

Brothers always follow events where sisters are. Whenever there is a gathering of a great number of sisters in one place, you're going to find some brothers looking to meet a nice sister. You'll also find men looking for sex. The first thing I saw after arriving at the hotel was hundreds of sisters dressed in their crimson-and-cream Delta colors. They had on red-and-white hats, scarves, shoes, and T-shirts, and it seemed like every sister had on her

Delta elephant symbol in some shape, form, or fashion. There were young, college-age sisters, along with quite a few middle-aged sisters, who seemed to be mentally back on campus. I also saw the stately, strong Delta Dears—the divas, the grandes dames of the largest black sorority in the country.

When I finally made my way through the crowd to the front desk, I could feel eyes all over me. I had on an all-black outfit, including my signature dark sunglasses. This is my favorite look because I look good and it makes me feel good.

After settling into my room, I wanted to explore the conference site to get a feel for the crowd—even listen in on some conversations, perhaps get some material for my speech. I wanted to see and be seen.

The first place I headed to was the huge lobby of the Sheraton hotel. Just off the lobby was a sitting area. A bar there served light food, and quite a few Deltas had set up camp, checking out the crowd, greeting their sisters, laughing, and eating. I caught some of them giving me that "I want to get to know him better" look when I walked in the room. I seemed to be one of only a handful of men there. I went to the bar and ordered a Bloody Mary.

I overheard a sister at one table say, "That is one good-looking brother right there." The other women at the table agreed, and one even gave her a high five. I turned and smiled.

I sat between two sisters at the bar who were not talking, just drinking. I smiled as I excused myself and sat down. The sister to my right smiled, and the other said hello. After I got my drink, I struck up a conversation with the bartender, an older white man. We talked about Baltimore and other light topics. When he left to make more drinks, I leaned over to the sister on my left and asked if she was here for the Delta conference. She said she was and went on to tell me what the conference was about, who was attending, and what her organization did.

The other sister joined our conversation, and after a while the three of us were talking, laughing, and having more drinks. I never told them who I was or that I would be speaking at their conference.

I asked them where the parties were and where all the single sisters were hanging out.

"You only looking for single sisters?" the sister to my left said, and started laughing.

"No, I'm looking for any sister who will treat me like a king," I said.

Both sisters started laughing, and I joined in. I was establishing a connection.

The sister on my right had to leave, but before doing so, she wrote her room number on a napkin and told me to give her a call if I wanted to hang out that night. I told her I would.

The other sister and I started talking about nothing. I turned my body to face her. I was on my third drink and feeling good. I asked if she was married and, if so, whether or not her husband had come to the conference with her. She told me she was single and from the D.C. area. She went on and on about the lack of good men in D.C. and said she was two seconds from giving up on ever finding a mate for life. She went on to say that most men were either gay, in jail, or on drugs, and she didn't have time for the nonsense. At the same time, her eyes were saying something else. I asked for her card or her room number. She opted for the room number and wrote it down on the back of my business card. I told her I had to leave, and as I stood up, I reached over and gave her a hug. She hugged me back. I told her I would call her later. "Maybe we could get together, and I could prove to you that there is at least one good man left," I said. She smiled. I smiled and walked away.

As I headed across the lobby, I noticed a long line of Deltas trying to get an elevator. I had to wait with the rest of them to get to my room on the eleventh floor. I worked my way through this sea of crimson and cream. I smiled and talked to those sisters I saw looking at me or who I thought were attractive. The line was not moving, because the Delta Dears were given first priority to get an elevator.

Back in the room, I got ready for my speech. I had changed into a gray suit and tie and was smelling good. I stopped again at the lobby bar, where there were twice as many women as earlier. I could not pass up this opportunity. I picked up a copy of *USA Today*, headed to a couch, sat down, and pretended to read. Across from me was a sister eating a sandwich. I looked at her and said, "I am starving. You know, you need to share that sandwich."

She said, "No way. I just got here, and I am hungry."

I told her that was no way to treat a brother. "Here I am in the middle of all these women, and I just want one to show me some love."

"I know you will get plenty of love from my sorors," she said, laughing.

I agreed with her and said I was looking forward to hanging out. I told her I had heard there was a special club called the Delta something or other where all the single sisters would be getting their party on.

"Yeah, you will be like a kid in a candy store at that spot," she said.

"No, not me. I just want to have a little fun while I'm away for the weekend."

I asked her if she would like to hang out with me that night. She said she liked to dance. I told her we could tear up the dance floor.

"I'm a nice brother, with no criminal record, I love my mother, and I take care of my kids," I told her.

She laughed and said, "Give me a call," as she wrote her cell number down on a napkin. It was time to get ready to speak. When I was being introduced, I looked into the audience for the sisters I had connected with. By the time I got to the podium, I had spotted a few.

"Good evening, ladies. My name is J. L. King, and I am here tonight to talk about why so many of our sisters are being infected with HIV. It's partly because of brothers who look like me and act like me. It's from brothers who like to have sex with women *and* men."

I could hear gasps in the audience. Most of these women would never have suspected that I was living a double life—especially not the ones I had gotten numbers from. I was the last person they wanted to see up there. I scared the hell out of many of the women that night and made quite a few very angry.

Afterward I was practically mobbed. Women were

telling me flat out that I was wrong. "I know my man, and there is no way he could possibly be on the DL." Another woman told me, "I'm married, and my husband would never do that to me. He is not gay!" Some sisters agreed that this behavior might exist, just not in their households.

While I understand the fear and denial, I cannot ignore the numbers that say that black heterosexual women are being disproportionately infected with HIV. Somebody is infecting them!

One sister asked me, "What am I supposed to do? Stop having sex?" Another said, "I want to get married and have children. How am I supposed to know if my man is not being honest with me? Should I stop trying to find Mr. Right?"

Another angry woman said, "Why don't men do something?! Why don't y'all take some responsibility? Why is it always on us?"

Men have not taken responsibility for this, and many never will. Women must take steps to save their own lives: Don't succumb to peer pressure from your friends, family, co-workers, or anybody who says you must have a man at any cost. Love yourself and have open discussions about sex with your potential mate. Keep your self-esteem and self-confidence up by any means necessary, and treat yourself well all the time. And develop some good close male friendships. They will get you far.

One of the first steps women can take in protecting themselves is to not be desperate to have a man in the first place. I know it sounds harsh, but far too many women define their self-worth by whether or not they have a man. It makes it easier for some men to get away with leading a double life.

Too many sisters get caught up in the game. They want to feel special, they want to be loved, they want to be held. They deserve to have all these things and more. Brothers will give them everything they want, make them feel like queens, and they will never suspect the ugly, hidden secret. It is important for a woman to value herself and always protect herself no matter what.

At one point I was dating this sister named Lisa. I had met her through some friends, who told me they had the perfect woman for me. She was a little overweight (they knew my love for shapely women) and very attractive. She was a bit insecure but had a great job and money and owned her home. We were set up on a date. Lisa had a beautiful personality, and we hit it off immediately. She loved to talk and loved children. She loved to laugh and knew how to make me laugh. She loved spoiling me and didn't hold anything back.

After a few months we started dating seriously. We were having sex on a regular basis, and she was becoming a part of my family. We were a couple. I was happy and looked forward to spending time with her. During this time we also attended family gatherings together.

One day I went to see her at her house. I knew it would not be a long visit, because I had someplace to go the next day, but I wanted to see her and get some. The sex we had was great. We would have sex and make love at the same time. Lisa might run a bath one night with a floating candle for us, and I would bring the takeout and we would eat, and I would spend the night holding her. Another night we might go straight to the bedroom—no foreplay needed. We had a very passionate relationship. Lisa never asked me to wear a condom, and I loved that. She allowed me to do her any way I wanted, and she made sure I knew that I was the best she had ever been with.

When I got to her house, she would often be waiting for me. We would always talk, and most of the time eat. But we would always end up in the bedroom. On this particular night it was a rush to the bedroom. I was in a selfish mood sexually. She knew it and didn't care. Afterward I showered and left.

I stopped at the gas station on the corner to fill up, and as I was pumping the gas, this smooth-looking brother about six feet two and 195 pounds walked through the station and said, " 'S'up."

I nodded at him and said, "'S'up."

He gave me a nod that said he liked what he was looking at. I nodded back.

We locked eyes as he continued to walk past me. He turned around and looked back.

"Got him!" I thought.

I nodded again and gave him another " 'S'up," which really said, "Look, bro, come on back and talk. We both know what's up."

He picked up on the nonverbal communication and came back toward my car. After some small talk we were on our way to his house. He told me he lived with his mother because his girl had put him out. We went in the back door and down the stairs to the basement, where he had a room. His space was beside the laundry room—just a mattress on the floor and a TV. I could tell he was down on his luck. He talked about not being able to find a job and needing to make some money so he could pay his child support. I told him right then that I was not paying to get with him.

"No problem," he said. "I was just sharing."

We started undressing, and there was no more reason

for conversation. I had told him before we got there that I was a total, 100 percent "top," meaning I did all the penetrating and I would not be penetrated. He said he was cool with that and that he could go either way.

After we finished, I put my clothes back on, gave him a twenty-dollar bill just because I wanted to, got his number, and booked. I called him from the car later and told him I wanted to see him the next time I was in the city. I then called my baby, Lisa.

Sadly, too many women are so desperate to have the perfect man that they do not ask questions, they don't do their homework, and they do not think about the fact that they are putting their lives in jeopardy by engaging in unprotected sex.

Society puts so much pressure on women to be in relationships, even if they have furthered their education and have a Ph.D., own their home, and have their own car. Even if a woman has a great career and has achieved a high level of success, she still has not made it if she doesn't have a man. Mothers and grandmothers pressure our women and young girls to get a man, always saying things like, "When are you going to bring a man home?" or "Girl, you're so pretty, why don't you have a man?" Or they will say, "You're almost forty years old. Your daddy and I want some grandkids." It's that type of pressure that has so many women throwing sexual precautions to the wind needlessly.

All the women's magazines talk about it: why a woman doesn't have a man and how to get one. Pressure.

The magazine covers scream at women: "Fifty Ways to Win a Man," "Top Ten Cities to Find a Man," "How to Please Your Man in Bed," "How to Give the Ultimate Orgasm to Your Man," "How to Communicate with Your Man," "Lose Twenty Pounds and Get a Man," and "Dye Your Hair Blond and Get a Man."

If you want a man, you have to please him. You have to change everything about yourself to keep him. Society puts all this pressure on women to get a man. And men like me know this.

When I go to clubs anywhere in the United States, I probably see ten women for each man. A lot of men who once upon a time could not buy a woman now have their pick and are attracting beautiful, smart, successful women. Men who aren't that attractive now have drop-dead-gorgeous wives. Men who are out of shape and have no job or income are married to beautiful doctors and lawyers. I look at them and say, "How in the world did you get that woman?!" It's because women want to have a man in their lives and that's the bottom line. A woman is told she is incomplete without a man.

Even the movies drive this point home. Many films have love stories that feature perfect romantic couples, and women want that. They see that and don't have it, and then they go home crying themselves to sleep or praying for that man to come and sweep them off their feet.

So when you meet a man who is on the DL, you don't even ask him about his sexual history. All you care about is that he's fine and has a good job and his own car. He can't possibly be gay. "He loves me" is all you say to yourself. You want to be held. You want to be loved and kissed. You want to be cared for. And your biological clock is ticking.

Women often ask me how they can avoid getting involved with a DL man. Sometimes I don't have the answers they want to hear. Nor do I have all of the answers. I can't tell them simply to ask, because if he's on the DL, he' going to lie.

Instead, I encourage women to restore sex to its rightful place as a sacred act. Women have tremendous power inherent in the choices they make about with whom they share intimacy and the terms by which they agree to do so. I encourage women to start out their relationships with men as friends, without having sex. Learn to listen to him, watch his habits, and get to know his friends. If there is something that doesn't feel right, or if she feels he's being secretive, she should tell him how she feels. Too often women ignore the inner voice that tries to give them an early warning signal.

Women should open up about their own sexual histories and expect that potential sexual partners do the same. Talk to him about his sexual habits and past sexual partners. Women should share how they feel about men who cheat, men who are bisexual, and men who are on the DL. She must let any prospective lover know that she's aware of the behavior and that she doesn't want to be involved with a man on the DL. And most important, she must make it clear that she practices safe sex, and tell him that she wants to get tested together so that she can have peace of mind and share intimacy more completely with him.

For women who are married or in a long-term relationship where condoms are no longer being used, I recommend that they get tested, and ask their mate to get tested without accusing him of being on the DL.

6

"OH, GOD!"

Being raised in the church from the first Sunday I was home from the hospital, I have always had a deep love and respect for the church, for prayer, and for the leaders of the church. I was taught that if you are a good person, respect others, say your prayers every night (to ask God for forgiveness and thank Him for His grace), obey your parents, and give God 10 percent of your earnings, then you will almost certainly have a place reserved for you in Heaven.

In my house my brother and I did not have a choice about whether or not we would go to church. We attended Sunday school and were active in everything, including holiday plays, youth choir, and usher board. We even went to vacation Bible school. The bad kids knew that Deacon and Mrs. King's boys were well behaved and were not to be picked on or messed with. Everybody knew that my mother would be in your face if you even looked at her two darlings.

We didn't cuss, and we feared God. We said our prayers over every meal. Every night, on bended knee, we said the Lord's Prayer. My father was at church meetings throughout the week. There were prayer meetings on Wednesday nights, deacon meetings on Thursdays, and men's choir rehearsals on Fridays. He was also active in maintaining the church, from cutting grass to doing odd jobs. Deacon King was a true church leader.

I have always had a clear understanding of my belief and love of God. I have never used His name in vain. I fear God. It is one of the reasons that I didn't smoke or drink while in high school. I was also a virgin until the day I got married. I would wait, and then do the right thing. I respect my elders. Even today I call men and women older than I am "sir" and "ma'am."

I have had some unbelievable blessings in my life, and I know without a shadow of a doubt that they were sent by God. There is no way I could have received the type of job promotions, growth opportunities, and many, many other blessings if it were not for God. I know that God's hands have been on my life, and He is always there to keep me from falling and continues to bless me.

As far as my sexual lifestyle goes, I used to pray and ask for His forgiveness every time I would sleep with a man. However, I have stopped saying that prayer. I now ask Him to continue to allow me to be the best person I can be. God knows what I am going to do before I do it. He knew me before I entered this world, so I no longer trip on what I did or do. I did not choose this. I know this desire is something I was born with and not something I learned or decided I would do. I have no control over these double desires. When I die and stand before my Father, I want Him to judge me based on how I loved and how I helped others.

The book *Conversations with God* by Neale Donald Walsh has provided me with 100 percent peace of mind about my life. In this publication God tells the author that He gives all of us free will to live our lives. He, God, doesn't intervene or make decisions for us. Because God has given us free will, He will not punish us for the decisions we make. That's comforting.

I question whether having sex with men and women is a sin. I think that abusing people who give you their bodies, minds, and souls by not being honest and true is a sin. I am thankful that I now know that. Yes, I was living in sin when I was lying and putting others at risk of death and destruction. Now that I give my sex partners a choice—free will—I feel I am no longer living in sin.

7

THE BLACK CHURCH

Do you not know that the wicked will not inherit the kingdom of God? Do not be deceived: Neither the sexually immoral nor idolaters nor adulterers nor male prostitutes nor homosexual offenders nor thieves nor the greedy nor drunkards nor slanderers nor swindlers will inherit the kingdom of God. —1 Corinthians 6:9–10

Greg, a forty-three-year-old bank officer from a major city, was the type of brother who used his looks to get attention from men. He worked out at local gyms and had the kind of body and face that brothers had a hard time *not* checking out. Greg was a total bottom—meaning he liked being submissive—and loved sex. He had been engaged to a beautiful woman but decided he would be happier not lying to women anymore, so he left her and decided to be upfront about his lifestyle. When I asked him how he identified his sexual orientation, he said, "A man, bro. No label. I'm not on the DL, I'm not gay, I'm not bisexual. I'm just me."

Greg's attitude toward labels is typical, but what was not typical about him was his desire to purge. He wanted to talk about one incident in particular that he's not proud of and is still grappling with: his sexual encounter with a man of the cloth.

"Many pastors preach from the pulpit against homo-sexuality," he said. "But some of them are just being hypocrites." Greg then told a graphic story about a sexual encounter he had with the pastor of his church.

Greg continued to attend church there, but later found out that the pastor was also having sex with one of the male associate ministers. Still, his sermons against homo-sexuality didn't end.

"In fact, he started preaching even more about the sub-ject," Greg said. "I would sit there and listen to him con-demn two men lying together, knowing the truth."

For many of us the church is the anchor of our lives. The black church has been a central place for people to seek sal-vation and acceptance. The church has been the place where most turn when there is no place else to turn. It was the black church that helped usher in the civil rights movement and provided much of the support to rid our nation of Jim

Crow laws. Many leaders of black churches throughout the country have been at the center of not only their churches but also the political scene.

National organizations like the Balm in Gilead in New York City provide education and training to churches that want to establish HIV/AIDS-prevention programs. The Balm in Gilead works with faith-based organizations to assist in fighting homophobia and other negative messages in the church.

However, on the issue of HIV/AIDS and the causes of the disease, the black church has often been sorely lacking, providing little or no comfort at all. It's as if the church were in denial. Few churches seriously address HIV and AIDS among their congregations. They are also unrealistic about the number of members living double lives.

When a sister approaches her minister about her husband who she suspects has been cheating on her—even if it is with a woman—he will often advise her to pray for her husband, go home, and stand by her man. Pastors need to understand that while prayer can conquer all and can change people, that sister is playing Russian roulette with her life until that brother actually changes.

Many ministers think they are making an impact through their sermons admonishing homosexuality. But for men who don't consider themselves homosexuals, that message simply isn't getting through. How many times have we heard the tired "God made Adam and Eve, not Adam and Steve" sermon? Preachers always want to take you to 1 Corinthians ("nor homosexual offenders . . . will inherit the kingdom of God") and the Book of Romans, where Paul says, "Men committed indecent acts with other men and received in themselves the due penalty for their perversions." Some churches even teach that HIV and AIDS are the "due penalty" for homosexual acts. They tell you how much God hates homosexuality. They tell you how you will go to hell, burn in the lake of fire for sexual immorality. What most churches won't do is take the Book of Romans a few more lines down to chapter 2, verse 1: "You, therefore, have no excuse, you who pass judgment on someone else, for whatever point you judge the other, you are condemning yourself."

This finger-pointing and judgment by the church and its leaders have not saved lives. They have turned people away from the very thing that may save their lives *and* their souls—God. The church leadership needs a new approach because the message of fire, brimstone, and damnation is not working. People need messages of prevention that acknowledge the reality that parishioners are having sex.

The black church has to deal with HIV/AIDS not so much from a biblical perspective as from a social perspective. I'm not saying forget the sin; I'm saying forget the condemnation, the finger-pointing, and the judging of others. Deal with the issues.

George McRae, pastor of Mount Tabor Missionary Baptist Church in Miami, Florida, has begun to help people heal spiritually. He received a call from a white chaplain at a local county hospital who told him about a ward in need of his help, a ward full of black men and women with AIDS.

McRae didn't run away when called; he came with arms wide open. His actions are chronicled in a February 14, 2002, *Wall Street Journal* article titled "One Black Church in Miami Takes a Rocky Journey to Confront AIDS." In this piece McRae's ministry is identified as having one of the most aggressive AIDS programs of any black church in the nation. It began when he visited this AIDS ward and was appalled by what he saw: men and women who had been locked out of their community, shunned by friends and family.

In *The Wall Street Journal* article Pastor McRae said, "It was embarrassing and painful, that someone from another community had to call me and show me how my own people were suffering. Every black church should have an AIDS ministry."

Pastor McRae told his congregation that they should stop thinking they were better or holier than the brother suffering from AIDS because he got the disease from homosexual sex. McRae also gave a speech, "The Black Church as Change Agent," at an AIDS conference in Atlanta. In his speech he claimed he could not condone homosexuality, because the Bible doesn't. He also stated that he doesn't reject gay people any more than he would an adulterer or a murderer. He said he was reaching out to people infected with the disease because God said He loves all of us.

At a time when AIDS is ravaging the African American community, the nation's black churches have been slow to respond. What McRae is doing in Miami should be commended and emulated throughout the nation.

Maybe some ministers are avoiding the topic because of shame and guilt for their actions.

I know a pastor in Chicago in his late sixties who had lived on the DL for forty years. He and his assistant pastor were lovers for more than twenty years. He is now trying to be an upstanding minister. He has retired from the DL community and has given up sex with men and women.

There are gospel conventions throughout the nation for churches. There is one for ushers, Sunday school departments, ministers, and music departments—which include choirs, musicians, and music directors. These events allow men to meet and to have sex while away from their hometowns. Many midnight concerts turn into affairs where brothers are cruising each other. I've been there, seen it, and done it.

You hear a lot of talk about Roman Catholic priests and their sexual misconduct. But no one is talking about what's going on in black churches. The black church has to stop the hypocrisy.

Black churches condemn homosexuality, while the pastor is carrying on an affair with Sister Jeanette, who sings in the choir. If you have an extramarital affair with a sister in the church, are you any more sinful than a man who is having an affair with one of the deacons? If you are doing drugs in the parking lot after church, are you more sinful than a man sleeping with the pastor? You have all types of categories or levels of sins. Why break this one out? The Bible talks about a whole lot of sins. The Bible even says, "If you know the good you ought to do and don't, you have sinned."

The church focuses on certain sins and blows them out of proportion. The pastor feels he has to give that "homosexuality is a sin" sermon once a month, because he sees so many gay men in his church, or gets pressured by his members to speak on it. Is that sermon going to change those men? No, all it's going to do is push men away from the church.

Ministers have an excellent opportunity to provide education, compassion, and understanding.

The black church must preach the truth and become a place where all men can come and hear the Word without feeling they will be judged or ostracized, regardless of their sexual orientation. It should be a place where sisters can depend on getting sound advice and be counseled to love and protect themselves *first*.

The church should provide comfort to single sisters as it encourages them to wait for the one God has chosen for them. A lot of large churches have singles ministries and offer outlets for their single members to socialize and meet under the umbrella of Christian love and standards.

Having grown up in the black church, I know all the good a church can offer the community it serves. I know the church could have an impact on how black people think about homosexuality. The church could start teaching love, not hate. The church could provide support systems for men who want and need help dealing with homosexual desires.

If we can't turn to our churches, where many of us grew up and to which many of us look as an extension of our families, then we will continue to live in denial, praying that God will forgive us and still allow us to enter into the gates of Heaven.

8

TO SERVE AND NOT PROTECT

When I was in the U.S. military stationed at a remote base overseas, there were very few African American men or women in the nearby town or on the base. On the weekends most of the brothers hung out in one another's dorm rooms. A few of the higher-ranked enlisted men lived off base. Most of them were involved with the local women, who were white.

Every soldier was assigned a higher-ranked member of the enlisted personnel to get oriented to military life, and Fore was my supervisor. He was twenty-seven years old and from the states, with a big-city attitude. He had been in the U.S. military for three years. My roommate and I were nineteen and twenty, respectively, so we looked up to him, as did a lot of young personnel. Many women on the base, both civilian and military, wanted him. You would hear the women talk about him and how good he looked. He was well built, with bowlegs and he was cocky. He was a player. And he was one of the few personnel who had his own car. He was the BMOB, big man on base.

Fore and I worked in the same office. We were not very close, but he would always ask me about my roommate, O. O. was from Upstate New York, and we hit it off real fast. We would spend lots of time together, talking mainly about our girlfriends back home.

O. would come to my office to pick me up for lunch, and in hindsight I realized that Fore was always checking out O., who said Fore reminded him of his uncle. Fore loved to drink, and I thought he was a part-time alcoholic. He was always at a military club getting drunk.

One Friday, Fore invited O. and me to his apartment off base. We had not been off base in a long time, so we jumped at the opportunity. He picked us up at the dorm and drove us to his apartment about twenty miles north of the base. When we got to his place, we unpacked, and he told me that I could have the couch and said O. could crash in his room. He had a king-size bed, big enough for both of them. We all went out to a hole-in-the-wall bar to do one of Fore's favorite activities—drink.

When we were ready to leave, I asked Fore to let me drive because he was drunk as usual. He agreed. As I was driving, I heard O. say, "Take your hands off me, man!" I asked O. what was going on, and he said that Fore kept grabbing him.

Back at the apartment we carried Fore to the bed, pulled off his clothes, and covered him up. O. and I talked for a few minutes before turning in. O. went to Fore's room, and I had my spot on the couch.

I wasn't asleep very long before I was awakened by the sound of moaning. I got up to see what was happening. The door of Fore's room was closed, and I could see from under the door that the lights were out. I heard moaning—from both Fore and O. I went back to the couch. A few minutes later the bedroom door opened, and someone came out. I pretended to be asleep. I could feel someone hovering over the couch to check on me, and then he headed to the bathroom, did whatever he had to do, and went back to the bedroom, closing the door behind him.

The next day I got up first. The door to Fore's room was still closed. I was tripping but didn't say anything to them. O. came out of the room first. He had on pants and no shirt. He asked me how I slept. I told him I slept like a baby. He said he fell right to sleep, too. Fore came out of the room about an hour later. We had breakfast, and then went to the city to do some sight-seeing. The entire day not a word was spoken about the night before. Not one single hint or look. I sat in the backseat, wondering about it myself. Did I dream what I saw and heard?

When we got back to the base, O. and I continued being friends and never had a conversation about what happened. But I know what happened, and I also know that things like that were happening more frequently than the military would ever admit. In fact, homosexual behavior is not only looked down on in the military; it's a punishable offense.

The armed forces have a policy called Don't Ask, Don't Tell, whereby the military cannot ask if a person is gay; nor does a person have to admit he is gay, but if he is found to be gay or is caught engaging in homosexual activity, he will be dishonorably discharged.

This rule has forced gay men and women out of the military even if they are qualified to serve their country. It has also forced many who are gay to live on the DL. The DL society in the military is among the most secret, because if even a hint of homosexuality gets out, you can be turned in, investigated, humiliated, and drummed out of the military. You risk a lot to allow your secret to get out. If you show any type of homosexuality, you can be questioned and marked. Everyone will avoid you, and the whispers and gossip will start. If you are not married or dating a female, you may even be asked point-blank by your fellow soldiers if you are a "fag."

Military personnel love to joke about gay people. They tease and verbally abuse anyone who even remotely acts like a "homo." But even with the threat of dishonorable discharge and shame, men and women still find a way to act on their desires.

While doing my research, I came across a young man named Kyle, who had been in the army for several years. He told me that when he enlisted, he knew he was attracted to men. He said he had "messed around" his entire life. Kyle had a girlfriend and, like so many young men who enter the military, had planned on getting married. But for this young man this plan was just a pretext.

"As a soldier, I really tried to keep my desires for men under cover," Kyle told me. "I tried to stay focused on my job and all that Uncle Sam offered me. But when I could no longer keep masturbating in my room, I ventured out to the local city to see what I could get into. I had heard about a park that gay men cruised. I overheard a couple of my army buddies talk about going over there and kicking some fag's ass. I had heard the rumors about soldiers who had gotten busted in the park and been dishonorably discharged. I knew the risk would be great, but I was willing to take that chance."

One weekend he changed into civilian clothes and headed for the city. He said he drove by the park, but he didn't see anyone. It was early. So he headed to the bus station.

"Back home you could always pick up a brother at the bus station," Kyle said. "You could find a hustler hanging around or someone homeless who was willing to have sex for a few dollars or to get off the streets for a few hours."

He didn't have any condoms. He said he was planning to pick some up at a local store just in case he got lucky. But he never made it. He went to the bus station, wearing his baseball cap pulled down low and a pair of dark glasses.

"I was not looking like a soldier," he said. "There were always a lot of men from the base in the city on the weekends, looking for women or trying to pick up a woman at one of the many local bars. I didn't want to be spotted."

At about eleven he parked his car. He looked out the window and saw a few brothers standing around.

"No one caught my eye, and I decided to wait," he said.

He figured he would get into something and return to

the base before anyone knew anything. After about an hour a brother walked out of the bus station door with a lit cigarette in his mouth. He looked thuggish. Kyle blew his horn to get the attention of the man, who looked and walked toward the car.

"I got out and said, ' 'S'up,' " Kyle said. "I asked him what was going on. He said nothing and that he was going to find a motel to crash at for the night. He was waiting on a MoneyGram from his girlfriend so he could get a ticket to California. I asked him if he wanted to take a ride. He said sure. He grabbed his duffel bag, threw it in the backseat, and jumped in."

They headed for a cheap motel, checked in, and went to the room. It was a tacky $19.99-a-night room with a raggedy regular-size bed, Kyle said. The man sat on the edge of the bed and fell back. Kyle sat in the chair and took off his boots. He turned on the TV and took off his shirt. Then he turned on the air conditioner.

Before long, both men were in the bed, naked. When they were done, they got dressed, grabbed something to eat, and checked on the dude's MoneyGram. After the dude got his money, Kyle dropped him off at the bus station to get his ticket to California.

"I didn't even think of what we did until later in the

week," Kyle said. "I let this man, a stranger, have sex with me without any protection. I didn't even think about the risk that I put myself in. I just prayed that it was going to be okay, and life went on."

But for many men on the DL in the military, life doesn't go on. For far too many the pressure of being on the DL outside the military and having to go even deeper under cover in the military can be too much to bear. All branches of the military have DL men. They serve their country and they need to be able to get the type of HIV/AIDS education that will have an impact on their behavior, even if the military refuses to accept homosexuality.

9

THE CRIMINAL JUSTICE SYSTEM

In the early 1990s I was the director of sales for the Greater Columbus Convention and Visitors Bureau. I was the first African American male to have this position in Columbus, Ohio. I traveled all over the country. I had an unlimited American Express corporate card, the finest clothes, fine women, *and* access to fine brothers when I was away on business.

People thought I was the perfect gentleman. Chivalry was not dead with me. Brothers looked up to me. Politicians loved me. Bringing so much new business to the Columbus hospitality industry, I was making the city millions of dollars.

This position required that I travel to key cities and

sell Columbus as a place to hold conventions and meetings. The convention business is lucrative. Cities can make billions from conventions alone. When I was appointed to the position, only a handful of brothers and sisters were working in this field on a national basis. As the clout of the black travel dollar became more respected, cities started hiring and appointing more African Americans in prominent positions to go after the minority market.

I walked away from all this to pursue my own business. I cashed in my 401(k), rented office space, bought computers, and hired a few people. I had no idea what it took to start and run a business. I thought my name alone would draw a lot of contracts for me, but it didn't. My money was gone in less than three months. I lost my condo and my car and filed for bankruptcy. Everyone turned his or her back on me. I was no longer "Mr. Columbus"; I was just a brother out there struggling to make a business work. I no longer had the reputation or the American Express corporate card.

At the midnight hour I had to pack up or sell everything I could and head back to Mama's house. As I was trying to put the pieces of my life back together, a friend of mine told me that the Ohio Department of Rehabilitation and Correction was seeking RFPs (requests for proposals) from independent companies to develop a prerelease employment program that would be offered to inmates six weeks prior to their release. During this month-and-a-half period we would provide basic life-education training. We offered them job-interviewing techniques, résumé-writing courses, and the like to assist these incarcerated men in their transition from the penal system back to "normal" society. The bottom line was to keep them employed and out of the system by any means possible.

For this contract I had to compete with some large employment-training companies and established nonprofit organizations that provided services to ex-offenders. I prayed to God, and as always He blessed me. I was awarded a thirty-five-thousand-dollar contract to work at the toughest maximum-security prison in Ohio. The prison inmate population was 90 percent black.

I showed up at the prison dressed to impress. By the end of my first six weeks, I had trained more than a hundred inmates a day. Later I would have a hundred inmates in the morning and another hundred in the afternoon. Once I had a third class of inmates in the evenings, because the state was releasing a lot of men that year. I was getting rave reviews. I came in with the right attitude. I wanted to motivate these men to believe that they, too, could be successful.

At my main office I hired a very handsome, masculine

brother as my clerk. His name was Muhammad. He, like so many other inmates, had rejected the Baptist faith and had begun studying with the Nation of Islam. He wore the Muslim head covering and prayed three times a day. He didn't eat swine and always carried his Koran. He was quiet and well spoken. He had a wife and a kid and often talked about getting out and being a good husband and father. He had graduated from college while incarcerated. He was ready for the world. He had big plans, and he shared them with me every day.

We worked side by side in my office. Muhammad had excellent office skills. He was also well versed in brother-to-brother relations. Men in prison are a whole other breed. They can be craftier, more cunning, and more manipulative than brothers on the street. They spend their days plotting, and nothing gets past them. In prison everything you do is watched. Men are constantly looking for a weakness, anything to gain an advantage that will lead to more jail "privileges" or an opportunity to blackmail.

Muhammad told me about many instances of this, including some he himself was involved in. He told me about another prison office situation he had worked in. He said he set this brother up from the very beginning. Muhammad was a good-looking man with a nice body, and he would use that to his advantage. He would do both subtle and blatant things—like making sure he timed his coming out of the shower with his boss's arrival. Because of overcrowded penal conditions, space was tight, and the offices were right next to the showers. It was Muhammad's belief that any man can "get got," as he would say. I didn't believe this at the time, but Muhammad was able to land his prey. And this led to his being able to use the phone from the office as much as he wanted, extort money from his boss, and have more freedom than is normally allowed in prison.

I knew a high-ranking brother who worked at another prison in Ohio. His wife was the secretary to the warden. He was busted for having sex with his inmate clients. His wife knew he was being investigated, but she kept her mouth shut, even when they escorted him out in handcuffs.

Although some prisons take steps to try to quell sex between workers and inmates, too many prisons simply turn their backs and do nothing. This alarming practice is creating another breed of HIV-positive men who could potentially infect women and other men upon their release.

The United States has the largest number of people under criminal-justice control of any nation in the Western world. At the end of 1999, 6.3 million people, or more than 3 percent of all adult residents in the United States, were under the control of the criminal-justice system.

According to the CDC, many inmates are at high risk of becoming infected with HIV, hepatitis, or STDs. Many others come to prison already infected. This is because of past and continued risky drug use (sharing syringes and other drug paraphernalia) and sexual behaviors (multiple sex partners, unprotected sex, and untreated STDs). Recent data show that HIV and AIDS rates among inmates are very high.

Conventional wisdom would hold that because prisons are separate from the community, the danger of spreading diseases should not increase. But more and more, people are recognizing that this is not the case. The recidivism rate is high, particularly in minority communities, with inmates constantly moving back and forth between corrections and the community.

Almost all prison inmates eventually return to their communities, which means that their high-risk behavior and its effects come with them into the community.

The problem is heightened because many prisons simply are not doing the job of protecting inmates. Only nineteen states test all entering inmates. The Federal Bureau of Prisons and three states test all inmates upon release, and the bureau and six states also randomly test inmates for HIV. This lack of testing is having a deadly effect on our communities.

In my home state of Ohio, from 1995 to 1999 the number of state and federal prisoners testing positive for HIV rose to nearly 25,800. *The Akron Beacon Journal*, a local Ohio paper, has made the link between the rise in HIV among inmates and the spread of the disease among black women.

A March 2002 Centers for Disease Control news update stated:

> It is no secret among Ohio health officials that HIV is spreading rapidly among black women. What seems to be a surprise is that there might be a connection between the numbers of black men cycling through the Ohio corrections system—a total of 112,284 men between the ages of 25 and 44 over the last decade—and the upsurge in infections among black women.

Prisons aren't dealing with the spread of HIV. Women waiting for their husbands and boyfriends to be released don't know that they may be waiting to be infected as well. Men are lying about their sexual activities in prison, and they pass the results of that behavior on to their women.

Donald was an inmate in a maximum-security prison in Ohio. He had been paroled after serving five years on a drug charge. He told me that while he was not a "fag" when he was locked up, he would let the fags suck his penis, and he even had sex with a couple of them when he was high (yes, weed and other drugs are available in prison). He didn't care who knew about his sexual activity inside. It was quite accepted. He had a crew of men he hung with, and all of them had a boy "sissy" on the side. And of course no one used condoms. They weren't available. In fact, they are considered contraband in prisons across the country.

But on the outside, Donald had a girlfriend or two. He considered himself quite a ladies' man. He never looked at his prison experience as homosexual. He looked at it as "survival."

"I did what I had to do," he said. "Five years is a long time."

Now, that's not to say that every man in prison is messing around with other men, because that's not true. I don't think women should shun a man—fearing he may like sex with men—just because the brother has been locked up. Some men do their time, don't mess around while in prison, come home, and are good husbands and boyfriends. Just because a man has been in prison doesn't make him want to have sex with men. That type of picture falls into what some of the professionals are saying, which is that all ex-offenders became infected while in prison.

Some men who are locked up were having sex with other men before they went to jail; they didn't just start when they entered. And some will continue to have sex with men when they are released. They are no different from the Wall Street brother living on the DL who is married, has children, and has a house in the Hamptons. The bottom line is they are both having sex with men and lying to their women about it.

Many health officials believe that inmates and ex-offenders are the main reason that women are getting infected with HIV. They have stated that the lack of safer-sex education behind prison walls causes at-risk behavior among inmates. There's even a thought that prison rape forces men to become men who have sex with men.

I do believe that prisons must take more responsibility for protecting these men from themselves. The majority of prisons throughout the country do not allow condom distribution. They feel that somehow they would be condoning sex between men. But the reality is these men are having sex, with or without condoms. And they will continue to have sex.

Some prisons have rules punishing men for any sexual activity. In the Ohio prison system, masturbating will get you put in the hole. Instead of making silly rules forbidding masturbation, prisons should encourage men to masturbate as a means to minimize the desire to have sex or rape other men.

One inmate, who was involved with men on the DL before he was locked up, told me he was afraid to participate in sexual activities because homosexuals are not liked or respected in the system, especially by the prison guards. Those who are openly gay, he said, seemed to have problems from both the guards and the inmates. He told me about seeing young men get raped because they were "too cute," and they didn't have anyone to watch out for them. He even said some of the guards or professional staff would be sexually involved with inmates on the DL.

Men get raped in prisons every day. But there is also a lot of consensual sex. The prison community shows the diverse sex roles that men play. There are openly gay men in prison who act like wives and prostitutes and get paid with cigarettes, drugs, or extra favors. There are men who have sex in the bathrooms and in their cells. It is about gratification. Sometimes it becomes about companionship. A brother doing life might set up house in prison with a gay inmate just to have someone. Should he not have the right to have this relationship? Can the system really stop him?

Condoms and safer-sex education should be part of the indoctrination process for an inmate.

Men are getting infected with HIV in prison. When they come out, they are infecting others because a lot don't tell their partners their status. They chalk up their experience to a prison "thing," or, like many DL men, they don't even think of that activity as homosexual. A lot of inmates and men in the general population believe that if they get oral sex, they're not gay. They believe that if they penetrate and don't get penetrated, they aren't gay. Men having sex with effeminate, openly gay men in prison often don't look at what they're doing as gay. He's the closest thing to a woman, and since they can't have a woman, they rationalize.

There is a big debate over whether inmates and ex-offenders are the main reason that women are getting infected with HIV. Some health officials have stated that the lack of safer-sex education behind prison walls causes at-risk behavior among inmates. Health agencies have issued reports stating that more education needs to be made available to inmates and to those who work within the system. I feel that the correctional system needs to have condoms available in all prison dorms and housing facilities. And when an inmate is released and assigned to a halfway house or is back on the street, there should be outreach—perhaps through the parole system—to keep word out there about the dangers of HIV and STDs and unprotected sex. Along with the drug tests given to these ex-offenders, an HIV test should be given.

Education is key. There are so many misconceptions about the spread of the virus. When I have done group discussions about HIV/AIDS in correctional facilities, men have argued that women are the guilty party. They believe that women are passing the disease. Or they have a conspiracy theory: the government is killing off black people with this man-made virus. This bad information spreads like wildfire in prisons, where conspiracy theories take a front seat to truth.

10

TALKING TO OUR YOUTH ABOUT SEX IS KEY

Frank, one of the many brothers I interviewed for this book, shared a story with me that to this day still chills me to my core. It is the story of a young man, Nigel, whom Frank was mentoring and treated like a little brother. He, like so many young men, was naive and ignorant of many of the dangers in this world.

Nigel was a very intelligent, attractive seventeen-year-old high-school student. He stood six feet three inches tall and weighed about 180 pounds. He had planned to attend Howard University in Washington, D.C., where he wanted to major in business and accounting.

Nigel was the only child of a single mother. His father had left when he was a baby. He and his mother were very close, but she was not overprotective. She had raised him to make good decisions, and she talked to him regularly about the facts of life. She prayed for him every night and in her heart was satisfied that her son was "covered by the blood of Jesus."

Nigel was not a troublemaker. He was focused on his goals after high school, was an excellent student, and was active in his church and community. He didn't get caught up with the latest fashions, hanging out, smoking weed, or making babies. Nigel was very popular in school, especially with the girls. But he had eyes only for Monica. She was a quiet, attractive girl with dark chocolate skin. Monica also had a smile that could light up a room. She was in the National Honor Society, and she was going to be a doctor, like her parents.

Nigel and Monica were in the same math class. They had the same friends, and they spent time together on the weekends. Monica's parents treated Nigel like their son, and Nigel's mother loved Monica. When he was with Monica, Nigel never tried anything physical, nor did he tell her how he felt about her. They were both virgins.

They'd talk for hours on the phone about school, music, and the latest gossip. When Nigel was hired part-time at a popular footwear store at the mall, he was excited because now he could get his sneakers at a discount while earning money for college. One day a man in his mid-thirties came into the store to buy some running shoes. He struck up a conversation with Nigel and asked if he was interested in doing some modeling. The brother told Nigel he was a photographer who took pictures for CD covers and clothing companies. The man gave Nigel his card and told Nigel to call if he was interested. When he told Nigel how much he could make modeling, Nigel was very interested.

The man set up an appointment with Nigel for a photo shoot. Nigel called his mentor, Frank, to tell him about his good fortune.

"My good looks might finally pay off," Nigel joked.

Frank told him he wanted to go with him. Something about the scenario made Frank's antennae go up. Nigel ultimately decided to go by himself. Frank didn't know he had gone until Nigel called him later that night, saying he had visited the man's studio and had posed for pictures. Nigel told Frank that the man was very nice and that they had talked a long time about photography.

The photographer was from Washington, D.C., and was up north attending to some family business. Without trying to sound like he was questioning the guy's intentions, Frank asked Nigel if the man was married or had a girlfriend. Nigel told him he didn't say anything about that but he did say he had two children. Nigel was clearly impressed, saying that this guy was a "playa." He had shown Nigel pictures of his SUV and of his brownstone in southeast D.C.—not too far from the Howard campus.

The photographer and Nigel made plans to get together later in the week to look at the pictures and go out for pizza. The photographer was going to meet him after work, then follow him to the restaurant. He asked Nigel to bring Monica and suggested that they double-date.

"When Nigel said he was going to ask Monica to go with him, I was cool with that," Frank said. "At least Nigel would be with Monica. However, knowing the cunningness of DL brothers, I knew this was all part of the trap. He wanted to imply that he had a girl, and he also wanted Monica to like him—which was one of the main ways he could spend time with Nigel without raising any suspicions."

Frank knew the game. He had played it many times himself. But he still didn't say anything.

"I just tried to stay on top of it by talking to Nigel every chance I got, although this became more difficult because I was traveling a lot."

Nigel and the photographer were spending a lot of time together. Nigel's mother had met him and liked him.

She thought the brother was a good, positive influence. She had approved of Nigel's going with him to D.C. for a long weekend under the guise of visiting Howard. While he'd applied and been accepted to the school, Nigel had never visited Howard, one of the best black colleges in the nation. Monica had been to D.C. the previous summer with her family, and all her talk about the city in part influenced Nigel's decision to attend the university. Monica planned to attend nearby Georgetown.

The trip was scheduled for a weekend that Frank was due on the West Coast. He wasn't going to see Nigel until after his trip. Frank called Nigel to tell him to be safe and said, "Don't do anything that would hurt your mama."

"I wanted to say more," Frank told me. "But I didn't."

When Nigel returned home, he and Frank had a chance to talk, and Frank wanted to know all about D.C.

Frank questioned Nigel about the sites he'd seen in D.C. and wanted to know everything he had done. Nigel told him the trip was great. He said he and the man went shopping in Georgetown and did all the normal tourist things. They also visited the Howard University campus, which Nigel said was beautiful. Nigel also said that one night they went to a restaurant and listened to some black folks read poetry.

"Then he said something that caused me concern," Frank said. "He said they slept in the same bed. He justified it by saying the photographer didn't have much furniture. That is all he said about it. I didn't ask any more questions."

Over the next several months Nigel and the photographer spent a lot of time together.

"When I finally met him, he seemed like a nice man," said Frank. "He was very well-mannered and seemingly straitlaced. He talked to me about Nigel with a great deal of concern and sincerity. He was like a father figure."

A couple of weeks later Frank got a call from Nigel at eleven in the evening, telling him that he was bleeding.

"Where?!" Frank asked, very afraid.

"From my butt," Nigel said.

Nigel told Frank that he had found blood on his shorts. Frank asked him how long he had been noticing the blood. Nigel didn't say anything for a long time. Then he said, "Since I left D.C."

Frank asked why he thought he was bleeding, making light of it by asking if he had had a big bowel movement. Nigel said he needed to talk to Frank face-to-face. Frank knew what Nigel was going to tell him. That night he couldn't sleep from worrying about the conversation they were going to have the next day.

"I left work early and waited for Nigel to drop by after school," said Frank. "He showed up at my place around four o'clock."

Nigel asked for something to drink and headed for Frank's kitchen. When he returned, Frank asked if he was still bleeding. Nigel said, "Not too much." He had put toilet paper in his underwear, so he wouldn't get blood on his pants. Frank asked him what was going on.

At first Nigel danced around the subject, but Frank asked him straight out, "Did that guy screw you?"

"I had to be direct because I knew he was not going to just tell me easily," said Frank. "His eyes started getting real watery."

"Yes," Nigel said in almost a whisper. He told Frank they had sex when he was in D.C. He said the photographer didn't ask him. "I wanted to do it," Nigel insisted.

As Nigel went on to explain what had happened, Frank asked if the photographer had used a condom. Nigel said he didn't know.

"The room was dark, and I wasn't really trying to look at what was going on," said Nigel.

Nigel told Frank that the brother kept asking if he wanted him to stop, but Nigel said no.

"You didn't know that I get down like that, did you?" Nigel asked Frank, who said he just stared at him.

"He said he had wanted to tell me but didn't think I would understand," said Frank.

Nigel didn't want anyone to know, especially at school and certainly not Monica. He was sitting on Frank's couch telling *him* about being on the DL. That was ironic. He had no clue whom he was talking to. He had no idea how much on the DL Frank was himself.

Frank urged him to take an HIV test and asked again if the brother had worn a condom. Nigel finally admitted that the photographer had ejaculated inside him. Frank said Nigel needed to have an HIV test and promised not to tell Nigel's mother or anyone what had happened.

This was the early 1990s, and Frank went with him to get the test and waited anxiously for the results.

"Weeks after the test, Nigel received a call at my house from the clinic, saying he needed to come in to get his results," said Frank.

When Nigel and Frank went to the clinic, the doctors told Nigel that his test had come back HIV positive and he had contracted the virus that causes AIDS. Nigel didn't know what that meant. He just looked at Frank, who turned and looked out the window so Nigel couldn't see his tears. On the way back to Frank's house, Frank asked if Nigel had heard from the photographer in D.C. Nigel said that they had spoken a couple of times and that he was now working in North Carolina.

"I asked Nigel for the photographer's number, because I needed to call him," said Frank. "I wanted the brother to know that he had given this young man—my little brother—the HIV virus. I wanted to give this man a piece of my mind."

Nigel asked Frank not to tell his mother. Frank said that it would be impossible to keep this from her and that he needed to talk to Monica, too. Shortly after Nigel came back from D.C., he convinced Monica to have sex with him. This was right before their senior prom. Frank felt Nigel might have had sex with Monica because he was attracted to men and needed to validate his "manhood." Nigel and Monica had not used a condom.

"He sat in my car, and for the first time he cried," said Frank. "We sat there with the radio on. I put my arm around him and let him cry. I was so angry—angry at myself for not warning him, angry at him for having unprotected sex with that brother *and* with Monica. And I was extremely angry at the brother from D.C."

Monica got tested, and the first test came back negative. However, she was tested again later, and the test came back positive. Monica is living with the virus today.

Her life and the life of her family have changed drastically.

Nigel eventually died. He never got to go to Howard University. He never got to live a full life. Nobody knew what Nigel died of except a small group of people. His family, especially his mother, did not want anybody to know he died from AIDS. According to the death notice, Nigel died from pneumonia. This happens all the time in the black community—we hide the truth. I guess people think it is better to tell a lie than to admit to an unpleasant truth.

The D.C. photographer was never reached.

"Whenever I called the number, I got a recording," Frank told me. "Eventually the phone was disconnected. He didn't show up at the funeral, and I don't really know if he ever contacted Nigel during his last days."

Whenever I think about Frank and Nigel's story, I am even more willing to expose the DL society. Who's responsible for this tragedy—was it his mentor; his mother; was it his father, who wasn't there; was it his high school, which perhaps didn't give safer-sex advice; or was it his church? There are so many single women—grandmothers, aunts, friends, sisters, and cousins—raising children. These women have to educate young men about men living on the DL, as well as help them become more aware and observant about protecting themselves.

I know many young men who bring friends with whom they are sexually active home to spend the night at Granny's house, and Granny is oblivious. She thinks it's nice her grandson has such a close friend. I have talked with men who told me they were raised by their aunt or grandmother and they had a room in the basement—something similar to their own private apartment. They would sneak their sex partners in at night, and no one knew what was going on.

I know of stories where single mothers let their sons go on a trip with the deacon or a man in the church.

"Let me take your son to play basketball or go fishing," Deacon Jones may say to Mama. She lets her son go, no questions asked, because she's happy this man is showing an interest in him. She's stressed out and working a lot, and she hopes this mentor will have a positive influence on her son. She may feel her son needs a father figure or positive male role model in his life.

Mothers and fathers, grandmothers and aunts, and other guardians have to school their sons before someone else does. We may talk to our children about sex. But that little talk—especially in the black community—must now change to include same-sex behavior.

We may give our sons condoms, but it's with a wink. We encourage them to have sex with women, proving their virility and manhood. We don't talk to them about having sex with a man. It's as if parents don't even want to consider the possibility that their son might have sexual feelings for guys.

A handful of the DL men I interviewed claimed to have gotten involved with youth organizations and mentoring programs in order to hook up with young men. I'm not saying that all men in these organizations are on the DL, but I am saying mothers *must* pay closer attention to the men their sons are spending time with. As I tell women all the time, "Get nosy!"

We prepare our precious sons for so many things in life, but we don't prepare them for what Nigel experienced. It's time for mothers and fathers to have a different kind of talk with their children. They also have to warn their daughters about young men living on the DL. I'm sure Monica never once suspected Nigel of having sex with a man; after all, he was a "virgin." But she should have insisted on his wearing a condom.

Mothers don't want to think about their daughters having sex. They may talk about it, and they may even talk about birth control, but they need to talk about the dangers of having unprotected sex. A woman is more likely to contract HIV from a man than to give him HIV. Even if she is on the Pill or using some other form of birth control, she is at high risk every time she allows a man to ejaculate inside her.

According to the Centers for Disease Control in 2002, HIV was the fifth-leading cause of death for Americans between the ages of twenty-five and forty-four. Among African American men ages thirty-five to forty-four, HIV infection is the leading cause of death. Among African American women ages twenty-five to thirty-four, it is the leading cause of death.

It's even scarier:

- Young Americans between the ages of thirteen and twenty-five are contracting HIV at a rate of two every hour.
- An estimated 250,000 young Americans are un-aware that they are infected with HIV.
- By the twelfth grade 65 percent of American youths have become sexually active, and one in five has had four or more sexual partners, according to a 2000 CDC survey.
- According to a five-year study of almost 3,500 gay and bisexual men ages fifteen to twenty-two in seven U.S. cities, 14 percent of young African American

men who have sex with men were infected with HIV, nearly four times the rate of their white counterparts.

• According to the CDC, young African Americans accounted for 56 percent of all HIV cases ever reported among thirteen- to twenty-four-year-olds in thirty-four areas with confidential HIV reporting in 2000.

Young people have so much to face in today's world. They need to know that their home is the one place where they can be themselves without being ostracized. There is so much pressure on them. They need to know that Mom and Dad, Grandma, or whoever their guardian is, will love them no matter what. We have to talk to our youth and make them feel comfortable so they will talk to us.

TOPS AND BOTTOMS

My research has shown me that a lot of married, DL men enjoy being penetrated. They are penetrating and enjoying the sensation of entering someone at home with their wife or girlfriend. When they have sex with a man, they're looking for something different. Of the DL men I've interviewed, many are bottoms.

A bottom is the "passive," or receptive, partner in anal sex. Some men refer to themselves as "total bottoms," because they prefer receptive sex only; this is sometimes a way of gaining the attention of total tops and men who otherwise consider themselves straight. Some men enjoy penetrative sex with women but experience receptive sex with men. The perception of bottom gay or DL men being soft and swishy can be far from the truth.

Masculine bottoms seek masculine DL tops and sometimes will forgo the use of condoms in order to secure sex with men who are in denial about their activities with men. To insist that the top use a condom is to jeopardize the opportunity to have sex with this man. Condoms make the top face the truth of what he is doing.

Some men go either way. They are called "versatile," because they can switch from being a top to a bottom. Many men who experience man-to-man sex for the first time will be a top, because that's what they're used to. But once they get into it, they may find that they also like to be penetrated. Most men are socialized to accept their role as someone who penetrates. If a brother meets a man who wants to penetrate him, he may think it only fair that they share in the act and penetrate each other during sex.

There are subgroups, such as versatile tops and versatile bottoms. In these instances it depends on the emotional depth of the relationship between the men. Versatile tops are penetrative during onetime experiences but will be receptive if several encounters occur with the same person. Versatile bottoms are receptive during onetime experiences but will penetrate if more contact results with the same person.

Some DL men like only oral sex. These men generally prefer to perform oral sex on men they hook up with and are not open to other sexual activities. Sometimes it is mutual—each partner performs oral sex on the other. Many times, however, it is nonreciprocal—one partner gives while the other enjoys it.

Some men engage in oral sex exclusively because they are both tops and won't bottom for each other. It's a way of getting off without having to compromise. Or perhaps they feel that oral sex is safer than anal sex. It is easier to initiate sexual relations with another man through oral contact, which is faster to engage in and is viewed as being less homosexual than anal penetration. Unattractive men often use oral sex as a way to seduce any man.

Oral sex is considered the surest way of getting another man involved in sex. Many men are introduced to the DL life through oral sex. Some heterosexual men, if sexually aroused, will allow a man to orally service him— if for no other reason than to satisfy his curiosity or see if a man really can give a better blow job than a woman.

Todd, one of the DL men I interviewed, told me how he seduced a heterosexual man with oral sex. He worked at the police department with Deon, and he had confided in Deon that he occasionally had encounters with men. Deon responded by telling Todd he was strictly into women and wasn't interested in being with men. One day while on a break, Todd showed Deon a book he was reading. While flipping through it, Deon came across a very erotic section describing a sex act between a man and a woman that really turned him on. After reading the section, Deon said he wished he could get his lady to do to him what the woman in the book was doing to her man.

He told Todd that his wife never wanted to perform oral sex on him, even though he loved doing it to her. His woman on the side wasn't very good at it; somehow she always managed to get her teeth involved. Todd saw this as an opening.

"Well, I know where you can get the best blow job of your life," he told Deon.

"Where?" Deon asked, his curiosity piqued.

Todd just looked at him and gave him a sheepish grin.

"Oh, hell no, man!" Deon said. "I told you I wasn't into that!"

Todd calmed him down and again told him it would be the best experience he would ever have. After a day or two of consideration Deon followed Todd home one afternoon after work. His curiosity got the best of him.

12

THE SIGNS

"How can I tell if my man is on the DL?" I have been asked this question a thousand times. It's a question that eats at the souls of women. Some want to know because they have always suspected a family member or coworker. Others want to know what they should be looking for in their man.

Before E. Lynn Harris's *Invisible Life*, most sisters had never heard of the type of man I describe in this book.

Some women don't want to know anything about this particular guy, like the older black woman I met in Jackson, Mississippi, who told me I didn't need to say stuff that would put black men in a more negative light. She, like many people in the black community, feels that brothers have enough to contend with and that they shouldn't have to defend themselves against allegations of being gay or on the DL, too.

One woman had another suggestion. After *USA Today* did an article on me and the DL phenomenon in 2001, she wrote a letter to the editor describing how she found out that her husband was sleeping with men. She wrote:

Dear Editor:

I recently read your story about men who have sex with men. This story sickened me and angered me. My ex-husband was a man who had sex with men, and I didn't find out until a good gay friend of mine told me. He said he had seen my husband at a gay bar in the city about twenty-five miles from where we lived.

I asked my friend if he would approach my husband the next time he saw him there. About a month later, my gay friend told me that he saw my husband sitting in his car outside of the gay club and went up to him and made a pass at him. He said that my husband eagerly accepted his offer and asked him to get in the car. My friend made up an excuse why he couldn't, but asked him for his number. My husband gave him a pager number (which I didn't know he had).

I confronted him about this, and he denied it. I had my friend come over one day while we were having dinner, and when he walked in, my husband almost choked.

My advice to women is get you a gay man and have him come on to your man, it works every time!

Ms. Recently Divorced

If you don't want to go to such lengths, some subtle signs may tip you off. Men communicate nonverbally; they often use their eyes. In many ways, the hookup happens as it does when men and women are attracted to each other.

Communication starts with eye contact—a prolonged stare, a quick look, a sharp cut of the eyes, or a look out of the corner of the eye. That three-second glance can be all it takes to make a connection, or at least for the vibe to be felt. That three-second look can say, "I like what I see," or "Are you interested in talking?" or "Pull over at the next gas station, let's talk." All the while, that man's woman might be sitting next to him in the car while he's making a connection with a dude.

If a sister has ever had a brother pull up next to her at a traffic light and give her the eye while her man is behind the wheel, she will know what I'm talking about. The brother will glance at you, then at your man to make sure he's not paying attention. You may smile, and he may wink at you. The same thing happens with a DL connection.

The word " 'S'up" is a popular greeting that can be exchanged sometimes by just a nod of the head. I saw a commercial recently that had brothers only giving the 'S'up nod. No words needed to be exchanged; it is a universal language used by black men of all sexual orientations and from all social, educational, and economic backgrounds. 'S'up, which means "hello," is shared between brothers. 'S'up can also carry an entire conversation between two DL men that sends the message "I am interested; are you?"

Nonverbal communication can happen anywhere. You could be walking hand in hand through the park with your man when another guy passes by and connects with him through body language and/or eye contact.

The signs are very subtle. Unless you lock your eyes on your man whenever he is around another man, it will be next to impossible for you to pick up everything he is communicating. You have to be careful not to overdo this. Becoming paranoid about every brother your man makes eye contact with could push a very good man away.

Some brothers make their connection with a hand-shake or a seemingly brotherly hug. A hug that is just a second too long will signal to the other brother that he is open to hooking up. Sometimes it is a key statement made in conversation that only another member of the DL society will pick up on. Sometimes the signs are so subtle that even men on the DL cannot tell if a brother is interested.

I was being asked questions about signs so much that I posted on my Web site a list of "The Top Questions Asked About the Down Low Behavior" with the question *How can I tell if my man is on the DL?* as the number one question.

I have been asked questions like "If a man enjoys having his ass played with is he gay?" "What if he has too many close male friends that I don't know?" "What if he isn't having sex with me often, or why is my man acting like he isn't sexually aroused by me?"

One sister wrote:

I am a single Black female currently dating. I'm always a little suspect of men who want to have anal sex with me. I figure if they do it to me, they will be willing to do it to anyone (male or female). I know anal sex is the big thing now, but I do not enjoy it and I am not afraid to let anyone know. Do you think that is a sign that a man is on the DL?

All these aspects of their man's behavior could be signs that he is on the DL, or they could mean something else. Maybe he enjoys having his women do nontraditional sexual play, or he is just not in the mood due to health reasons, stress, or lack of interest. A woman should not automatically label her man "on the DL" when his actions change.

The first thing I want to say to women who are seeking DL signs or behavior traits is that not every black man is on the DL. Not every black man in your life is on the DL.

Some DL men are so good at hiding their "hookup" skills that even when one is making those sexual connections when you are with him, you will not see it. Most DL men make connections away from the home. Maybe he will meet another man while just shopping at the mall, or while walking the dog. You cannot be with him twenty-four hours a day. You don't always have access to his e-mail accounts or his phone calls, and you don't always know if he is where he tells you he is.

Some will lead you to think that they have another woman. Men know that women will try and compete with other women. And some women don't care if her man has another woman in his life. As long as he brings home the check, and takes care of her needs, he can do whatever he wants. I have asked sisters, "How many of you would have that same attitude if the other woman were a man? Would you still care, and just want the check?"

Some women know their man has sex with men. They have either caught him, found proof, or been told by reliable sources. But they don't care. They continue on with the front to save face, or for the children.

I also want to make sure that I am clear when I say not all black men are living a double life, a double lie. Gay and DL men approach many straight men every day. And they choose not to have sex with another man. I beg women not to indict all brothers because of what I am saying about one group of men. All men need to understand this behavior in order to provide education to their families, but not all men are on the DL. I would hope that my daughter meets one good non-DL brother who will love her and give her the type of relationship that every woman wants and deserves.

I don't have a "sure list of signs" that will give women the answers that they seek. Women can hire a private investigation company or get a very masculine-acting and -looking gay man and have him approach their man. But, most important, they should strive to have a relationship where they can talk freely about sex, where they can have the power of choice through open, honest discussion.

The first thing women can do for themselves is open their minds to the possibility that their man might be interested in other men. I'm not saying that a woman should ask her man or confront him without cause, because that is asking for trouble—especially if he is not out there messing around on her.

Women have a powerful weapon against men living on the DL (or men who are cheating and scheming, period): their intuition. Many women have a sixth sense, an inner voice, and they are almost never wrong about things when it tweaks them. Women know deep inside when something's not right. They may not be able to put their finger on it. They may not be able to identify it. They may not have proof. But when a woman gets that little feeling inside, when that little voice tells her, "Something ain't right," she has to listen.

A DL man's first, last, and only line of defense, as I've said many times, is denial. He will lie, lie, lie, deny, deny, deny. After a woman's intuition taps her on the shoulder about him, she has to start playing detective to know for sure. She can't just approach her man and ask, "Baby, are you fooling around with another man?" His response will probably be something like "Why would I want a man when I have you?" or "That's nasty!" or he may get belligerent and tell her, "Why don't you stop tripping! What's the matter with you?!"

A woman has to be very careful about accusing her man if he's guilty. But she has to be especially careful if he's *not* guilty. She stands to lose a good man by doing something like that.

In addition to heeding her intuition, a woman can watch for a few signs. Is her man overly homophobic? If he is, watch him. Any man who *always* talks about "fags" or gets violent if any gay men are around or constantly bashes any and everything gay falls under the category of protesting too much. If a man is straight, there is no reason for him to feel threatened by a gay man. This kind of reaction usually is a result of not wanting to be found out. He goes to the opposite extreme in an attempt to prove that he can't possibly be gay. If he talks about it too much, get nosy.

A woman should also keep up with her man's comings and goings. A lot of DL men know how consumed their women are with the home, working, and participating in church and other social functions. They know how busy their women are, and therefore they know what they can get away with. A man knows his woman's schedule, and he will work his sex with men around that. A woman should know her man's schedule, too. And a woman shouldn't be so predictable. Drop in on him at work and take him to lunch one day out of the blue. Come home early from work one day; surprise him. It is more difficult for a man to get away with DL activity if his lady doesn't have a set routine.

When I was living a double life, lying to my women, I would and could do things without thinking about whether my woman was in tune with me, because I knew her schedule. When I was married, I was always home for dinner. I never canceled important events that my wife and I were scheduled to attend. I was home every night in bed with her. We made passionate love often. I told her I loved her. I hung out with her brothers, and her parents and friends loved me.

Even with other women after my divorce, I would pick up on how busy my lady was and work around her schedule. Throughout the relationship I would give her everything she could want or expect from me. When she became comfortable with the relationship and I had passed the "test," I would get even bolder with my outside sexual activity. I could do practically whatever I wanted and not fear getting caught. She was getting what she wanted and thought she needed, and I was doing what I wanted without raising any suspicions.

I'm not saying a woman should question all her man's friends. I'm just saying she should pay attention, watch, listen, and heed her intuition. How do her man and his friends interact? Has she ever walked into a room with them alone and felt a funny vibe?

Often women ignore that gut feeling because they don't want to know the truth. Maybe a woman's life is very comfortable; she so loves her lifestyle, the car her man has bought her, the house, the "status" he has afforded her, that even when confronted with that feeling, she may ignore it. She may not want to "rock the boat" or put her lifestyle in jeopardy.

Sometimes it is easier not to accept things that are hurtful and painful. My friend Renée shares her story about walking in on her ex-husband on the living room floor with his close friend—whom her children called "Uncle Bob"—but because she did not have a job, enough education, or family support she walked out of the room, and never said a word to her husband about what she saw. She was trapped, and until she could pull out of the relationship and leave, she was forced to smile and act like the perfect wife. One sister shared with me that she knew her man was having sex with men, but thought it was something that he would get over, and she could not leave him. Her love for him would get her through it. She was praying for him, knowing that God would change him.

Many sisters stay with men because they have no way out. I see young sisters who have two or three baby daddies—and sisters in love with men who are locked up; and when they are released, these men go back home to women who have only one thing in mind . . . *My man is home.*

If a woman loves herself, and knows she can do better, then she should do what is right for her. She should make sure that her choice is well informed when it comes to exposing herself to risky behavior that could have an impact on her life. She should make sure it's her choice, and not his.

13

DL BEHAVIOR TYPES

B ased on my research, conducting DL focus groups, and having personal relationships with DL men around the country, I have come up with a few DL behaviors. I have named each behavior based on background, age, region, lifestyle, and education.

I feel it is important that women understand the different personality types as they relate to the way these men act when they are on the DL. By understanding some of these behaviors, maybe women will be able to recognize them and make the right decisions and choices.

In this chapter I will introduce you to the Mature Brother, the Thug Brother, the Professional Brother, the "I Have a Wife/Girlfriend" Brother, and the "I'm Just Curious" Brother. When I talk about these five in my workshops, I have had women tell me that I have described every man in our communities. And that is my point; DL men are part of the daily lives of all of us. DL men don't stand out; they can't be picked out in a line-up or even if they are standing right next to you.

The Mature Brother

The Mature Brother has reached a point in his life where he has fine-tuned the skills to hide his DL behavior. He is experienced and has years of moving between both worlds. He knows how to get what he wants and keep what he has. He will not bring his two needs together. Some mature DL men will use their money, position, and access both to keep their wife satisfied and to get men for sex. I know some mature DL men who have adult children and grandchildren, and even a few with great-grandchildren. Many are financially independent, active in their communities, and hold powerful jobs.

This brother will take occasional risks to satisfy his sexual desires for male-to-male sex. You can find these men cruising parks and bookstores, hiring male escorts, or picking up street hustlers. Such a man knows that his wife doesn't have a clue about his DL lifestyle. His double sexual activities are kept far away from the home and family.

Since this life is a secret, being away from home, out-of-town, is the preferred way to explore their freak-on.

There are organizations and clubs in cities that cater to DL professional men, from private gentlemen's clubs to secret gatherings. There are mature men who understand the importance of keeping this hidden part of their life "on the down low."

Melvin, the man my wife caught me with, was the perfect example of a mature DL man. He was my DL mentor, and taught me how to have both men and women.

The Thug Brother

If you watch music videos, you see that the roughneck is the new sex symbol; he's the one getting all the girls. These days, even college-educated, upper-middle-class brothers try to be thugs to get women.

Likewise, some gay men take on the roughneck personality, because they know this is the calling card to attract men. In many cities organized sex parties are given just for these hardcore types and the brothers who want access to them.

The Thug Brother, or "homo-thug," is generally between the ages of eighteen and twenty-eight. You may see him downtown standing at the bus stop or train station, strolling in the mall, or walking or riding around with his boys. You will also find him on college campuses.

He always wears the latest urban gear—sagging pants, head rag, the latest sneakers and/or Timberlands (a must), and jewelry. He might have braids or dreads or sport a baldie. He loves to ride around with his partners, music pumping.

This brother could have several children by different women. He sometimes lives with his mother, one or all of his girlfriends, his homies, or his grandmother—any place he can comfortably lay his head.

He can be expensive and require undivided attention when he wants it. He associates everything with his sexuality. He's been beaten down by his experiences. He sees old-school methods—getting an education, working nine to five, being responsible—as a bad fit for him. He feels limited to the life he knows but will exploit that life for all it's worth. Sex appeal is his power, his voice.

He has most likely been to the health clinic, because at some point he has picked up an STD. He sees that as no big deal. He has little knowledge of the impact of HIV on the black community, because he doesn't read—neither newspapers nor reports—nor does he have conversations about it. He doesn't consider his sexual actions anything more than getting off. It is all part of the hustle.

In a June 6, 2001, *Village Voice* article titled "The Great Down-Low Debate: A New Black Sexual Identity May Be an Incubator for AIDS," Kai Wright explores this issue. In his opening paragraph he talks about how the comedian Richard Pryor used to do a bit where he joked about "fucking the faggot." "He wasn't declaring himself gay, far from it, and no one listening assumed as much. He was just admitting that he could get off by screwing another guy," Wright explains.

Wright also shares the story of Tevin, a hip-hopper described as "a lady's dream" and "also the Don Juan fantasy of a certain group of men: guys who live 'on the down low,' or DL." Wright quotes Tevin as saying, "I like girls. I have a girl. But every once in a while, 'cause women can be very stressful, I might chill with a dude. And it's just having fun. If something pops off, it pops off. Give each other a pound and meet up later."

Tevin is a typical Thug Brother. If he likes and trusts you, he will talk about his dreams of becoming an entertainer—one of the avenues left open to brothers like this. The Thug Brother may also tell you how he'd love to leave the city for bigger and better opportunities.

The Professional Brother

Meet Mr. On the Fast Track to Success in Corporate America—the Professional Brother on the DL. This brother has an education, and he is living the American dream. He is in a professional position or a high-ranking government job. He volunteers with social organizations or serves as a mentor or tutor.

He works out at the gym. You may also find him at trendy shops and festivals on the weekend or sitting in a coffeehouse with a young lady. He has season tickets to the theater and a ton of frequent-flier miles and flies business or first class. He is always dressed very *GQ*. He takes pride in his looks. He is a metrosexual, the latest label for men who care about their looks and image. He is articulate, speaks excellent English, and can be arrogant because of his status. He has all the trappings of success—from the platinum credit cards to the BMW. He owns his home and vacations in all the popular locations around the world. He is well connected and knows people. He has no criminal record and no drug habits and for the most part lives a decent and straightforward life.

This brother is the ideal man for a lot of women on the same track he is on. He would never date below his level;

status is a paramount concern. He admires successful women. He will date outside his race and can't understand why black women look at him with an attitude when he is out with a woman of another race, especially a white woman.

He is close to his parents and tries to have dinner with them on Sundays. He is a mother's boy and his family's pride and joy. He has always been an overachiever and understands the importance of getting a good education.

He will admit to women that he is in touch with his feminine side; he knows women like to hear that. He reads the latest issues of *Essence* and other popular magazines that provide in-depth information about women's issues. He is the type of man a woman can take home and her family will love. He brings her flowers, takes her to dinner, and opens the car door. He is the perfect gentleman.

His hunting ground for men is almost exclusively within his circle. He meets brothers at professional events, fund-raisers, professional conferences, and through his network of DL brothers across the United States. He will search the Internet for men and make contacts using his DL identity. If pressed, however, he will drive to adult bookstores and parks looking for men. He won't make the first move, but if the eye connection is made, he will make his move. He will take risks, if he is pressed. And he doesn't mind paying a hustler for sex.

This professional DL brother has sex with brothers within his professional community. He develops sexual relationships with his workout friends, fellow church members, and other professionals. The professional DL man may have more than one male sex partner. His high self-esteem (self-absorption) and his love of self make him feel like he is God's gift to everybody and that he is always in control—an important recurring theme.

In his public life this brother sometimes prefers white women over black women. White women don't ask questions. They figure if their man is doing something that seems odd, it must be a "black thing," and they don't pursue it any further. Some of these brothers are so caught up with their status that they feel white women are more on their level, mentally and financially, and will provide them with comfort zones to have sex with men without the drama and hassles.

This brother will maintain his DL lifestyle even after he has settled into a serious and permanent relationship with a woman. He will provide her with a home, a good income, children, and other distractions while he creeps with men. He will tend to have safer sex and may take an HIV test every time he has sex with a man. However, because of his strong sex drive, he is always in a state of denial regarding his risky sexual behavior with men.

I met Dr. Jones after answering a personal ad he had placed in a local newspaper. He was a specialist in cancer treatment and had established several successful clinics throughout the United States. He was a thirty-five-year-old millionaire.

We met at a nice restaurant, and there was an instant sexual attraction. We ended up back at his home. When we pulled into his driveway, I was overwhelmed by the house, grounds, and many cars parked there. At first I thought he had company. In fact, it looked as if he were having a very large party from all the cars. He had told me he lived alone and, because of the type of work he did, had little to no social life.

We sat in the great room of his very large and well-furnished home. He offered me a brandy. We then headed to the second level of the house because he wanted to get "started." He took the lead, bringing me to a bedroom he wanted to use—not the master suite. We used a guest room. We had small talk as we undressed. He told me that he was engaged to be married in the fall and that his girl lived in Michigan. She was also a physician. I asked if he did a lot of this type of sex. He said yes, that he would place personal ads for men and that that was his only way to find male partners.

We had sex, and he asked me to leave immediately after we finished. He was a very cold individual. He obviously didn't like that he had just had sex with a man. His attitude toward me was negative, and he wanted me out of his house. As I was leaving, he gave me his card and asked me to call him. I was surprised because of how he was acting. He didn't even look at me, just handed me the card and closed the door behind me.

Later that week he called and asked if I wanted to go away with him. He had planned a trip to the islands and didn't want to go alone. It would be a seven-day cruise out of Miami. He wanted my company. He was clear that he wasn't interested in sex, but he wanted someone to hang out with. I asked him, "Why don't you take your fiancée?" He told me she could not get away. Plus, he wanted to go with me, not her.

The thing between us lasted off and on for six months.

The "I Have a Wife/Girlfriend" Brother

This brother is so undercover, so on the DL, that he will not approach men, but he will stare and make sure he gets the attention of the men to whom he is attracted. To satisfy his need for sex with men, he will place ads on the Internet and depend on his handful of DL friends to hook him up. He will go outside his hometown and step out of his comfort zone by going to an adult bookstore or maybe driving around a gay bar—never going in. He may drive around and around until he sees another brother. He might even start a conversation with this brother. But if he's not sure, he won't go any further.

What makes him one of the most dangerous types to women is that he appears to be the perfect family man. His limited access to men and his strong desire to have sex with them cause him to act irrationally and unsafely. Sex with this man is about instant, desperate gratification. He doesn't have a lot of time for establishing relationships; he only wants to get off sexually and then get back to his comfort zone.

Once he meets a brother he is comfortable with and a connection is made, he will be loyal to this one man. He will invite this man to join his circle of friends and family. He will introduce his "friend" to his wife, girlfriend, friends, and family members. He will introduce the "new friend" as a coworker or pool-playing buddy. He will tell his male lover that his wife doesn't understand him and that they do not have sex. He may even say he is going to leave his wife once the children are grown and out of the house. He will also use the excuse that his wife won't give him oral sex or that his sexual needs are more than his wife or girlfriend can handle. He will tell his dude that he has always wanted to be with another man and finds nothing wrong with having sex with men.

The "I'm Just Curious" Brother

The "I'm Just Curious" Brother wants to pursue his curiosity about being with a man. He's intrigued but not fully sure if it's a road he wants to travel. He will not only fantasize about acting on his desires but also take risks to put himself in a position to be picked up. He is the only one of the five types of DL brothers I've met who will go to a local gay bar, party, or event.

If he's married, he might talk, seemingly innocently or jokingly, to his wife about his desires to be with a man. He will often prime that discussion by asking her how she feels about a threesome with another woman. This tactic will open the conversation for him so he can see where his wife is with the idea of his being with a man. He will lead her to make the suggestion of this kind of threesome. If he can get her to agree on the threesome, then in his mind he has the green light to go after a man. However, when he finds him, he will not include his wife. In his mind she is okay with this; it's not cheating, because he's "cleared it."

If asked, the bi-curious man will admit he has always wondered what it would be like to be with a man; this is his way to explore potential opportunities. He's a little more on the edge, because his curiosity often takes control of everything. It leads him into areas that his experience and logic would steer him away from. Then again, he may start from a place that leaves him oblivious of potential consequences or that gives him a mind-set of invincibility. Either way, he is more willing to operate on the edge of discovery than many other DL types—that is, before the reality of being discovered hits him in the face.

I haven't had much personal contact with bi-curious men, but a friend of mine, Andrew, shared one of his experiences. He said he met D. on January 21, 2001, after checking out the alt.binaries.pictures.erotica.black.male newsgroup, as he does regularly. He was looking for pictures of naked brothers when he spotted a listing by a twenty-nine-year-old Los Angeles area police officer. There was a nude picture of this brother, whose face was shielded by a police hat. He had a Web address attached to the photo.

My friend Andrew, who's gay but not out, worked for the LAPD and had to check out this site.

"I generally never visit sites advertised in a newsgroup, because they are usually full of viruses and Trojan horses," Andrew said. "I went to the site, and the pictures of this brother were off the hook. I downloaded the pictures and sent the brother an e-mail telling him that I enjoyed them and wished him good luck."

After twenty minutes Andrew received an e-mail from D. They exchanged e-mails every day, often three times a day. They talked about how D. was struggling with his sexuality. He was married, and he had known he was bisexual all his life. He said he was comfortable knowing he was bisexual, but he never acted on the feelings. Because of his exceptional physique, he was always being approached by men at the gym. He had never acted on their advances, because he didn't want to get involved in one-night stands with men. He wanted to develop a friendship, a real relationship with a man. His twenties were uneventful. A couple of his friends did come on to him, but he repressed his sexual desire for men at that point. He also did not have sexual interest in his friends.

He found a woman he knew he could be faithful to, and he married her, confident he wouldn't have to worry about being with a man. He posted these nude pictures of himself as a means of releasing the pressure that, he said, was building up in him.

"I found it strange that a heterosexual man would post nude pictures of himself on-line and advertise it in a news-group frequented by homosexual men," Andrew said. "But I made it my business to become his friend. I positioned myself as his mentor. I realized it was only a matter of time before he would have sex with a man. I decided to educate the brother, so that if he did meet someone, he would know how to determine if that man was worth risking his marriage, career, and health over. Since I was not an Adonis like he was, I never thought I would have a chance of sleeping with him myself."

Andrew told D. how manipulative and deceitful some brothers could be. He warned him to be careful about sharing personal information—that he could get seriously hurt out there. He told him that some men won't think of him, his wife, his health, his children, or his career. They will think of him as a piece of prime beef, an opportunity to turn out a straight brother and brag about it to their friends. Andrew told him he could fall victim to a situation where money would be demanded to protect his secret.

Eventually Andrew and D. met in person.

"I didn't know his name, his phone number, or his address. All I had was a Yahoo e-mail address and a fake screen name," Andrew said. "I didn't even know what he looked like. We were meeting at a mall, and all he said was that he would be wearing a red baseball cap. I spotted him and that body before I noticed the cap. He was just as gorgeous in person as he was in his picture. His facial good looks rivaled his body."

They talked at the mall, and then went back to Andrew's place. Two brothers sitting in a car at the mall would seem suspicious and attract attention. When they got to Andrew's place, they talked openly about D.'s feelings of bisexuality and the emotional roller coaster he had been going through for years. Andrew offered him a massage. D. agreed.

"I love giving deep-tissue massages to brothers, mainly because it is a non-penetrative way for me to connect with them on a deep level," Andrew said. "I also enjoy the challenge of massaging a well-developed muscular body. Most brothers have never had a massage, and it can really break a man down when done well."

Nothing sexual happened, but Andrew opened the door, awakening something in D. When D. got home, he immediately e-mailed Andrew, telling him he hadn't wanted to leave. He confessed that he felt aroused and comfortable. He asked if he could experience a few things with Andrew the next time he came over. Andrew agreed.

"I basically had a dream come true," said Andrew. "I was in awe of his body, and I had free rein over it."

The next time D. visited Andrew, they had sex. But D. didn't seem into it.

"I pride myself on making sure a man is thoroughly pleased," said Andrew. "But he was stiff as a board and nervous. There was no emotion and no movement from him. I realized that everything he had told me about himself and his marriage (that he had never cheated on his wife or been with a man) was true. He was scared of everything I was doing to him. I ended up jacking him off."

D. left and e-mailed Andrew the next day, expressing thanks for allowing him to experience man-to-man sex in a comfortable environment.

The next time D. came over, they had anal sex.

"D. was unsure of himself," said Andrew. "It was the first time since being married that he had slept with anyone besides his wife, and it showed. Before we had sex, he demanded HIV test results, and I had the paperwork showing I was STD free. The papers were less than a month old. We used a condom. And when we were done, his face told me all I needed to know—he was in total shock over what he had done. As for me, I had an incredible sense of guilt, because I knew that should his wife discover this, his marriage and family would be devastated."

D. wrote Andrew the next day and said he had had the

most peaceful sleep in years. He was completely at peace with who he was. He felt whole as a man.

They became regular sex buddies, and their friendship deepened. But D. eventually wanted to keep his marriage, and he and his wife had a baby. D. and Andrew cut off the sexual part of their relationship but remained friends.

14

MAKING CONNECTIONS ON THE DL

DL brotha seeking other DL brothas for regular hookups. You are discreet, have your own place, be a freak, and not clockable. I am versatile, hung, a freak, and very masculine. I am only available from 9 A.M.–5 P.M. because of my family situation. Get back with me and no games. —Ondalow

When I was on the DL, the World Wide Web was better than hitting the Powerball lottery. I was like a hungry man who had just discovered a free all-you-can-eat buffet. And I took advantage of it, twenty-four hours a day, seven days per week. I lived online, looking and searching for other DL brothers who wanted to make sexual connections. And I found that there were many black men who just like me were discreet and on the down low, brothers who were looking for that sexual fix by any means necessary. All of the five behavior types of brothers that I describe in Chapter 13 could be found on the Net on Web sites, in chat rooms, and in personal ads. Whatever you wanted, it could be found on the Net.

When I first discovered the way that the Web could provide me with men without my leaving the comforts of home, I became hooked. All of my free time, and time that should have been used for more productive activities, was spent online looking for sex. At the click of a button, I could meet men, and as long as I was home alone, nobody would know.

My first online personal ad was simple, but as I read other ads posted by DL brothers, my ads became more creative. I worded my ads to attract real DL brothers, not gay men.

In one of my earlier ads, I wrote:

Attractive black male seeking other attractive black males on the serious low. Not looking for anything but sex. If you into women, contact me today.

Within days of placing the ad, I received many replies. Brothers from all over the country were hitting me back with their stats, and some included pictures. I didn't know at that time that brothers use other men's pictures they steal from Web sites featuring naked black men. I picked and chose those who had that masculine look, and their messages were what I wanted to hear.

I made a couple of contacts with men who lived in my city or within driving distance, or were willing to travel. I also placed at the top of my contact list those who told me they were married or had women.

I started communicating regularly with a brother in Los Angeles. I lived in Ohio, but the strong sexual vibe and conversations made the distance moot. We vibed, and because he was so far away it was easy for me to let my guard down. I was more open with who I was because he was too far away to cause me any problems. We met when he had had enough of the long-distance affair. The power of sex will make a man do anything. He told me that he'd convinced his wife that he had to attend a conference in Ohio. We spent the weekend having sex, and then he went back L.A. I'm sure that I was not the only Internet hookup he had traveled to meet. I also met an NBA player who had an ad that described himself as the "DL Athletic." He always wanted me to come and meet him wherever the team was playing. He was very comfortable with me even when we hung out. The women around the players had eyes only for the players, not their friends. I have seen many women agree to sex just because the brother was a professional ballplayer. I also know that many professional and nonprofessional sports players have men on the side. Just like with women, many have a man in every city.

Looking for all you DL men who can appreciate class and tired of dealing with boys. Roll the dice, you might win. Your turn. —TheOne4U

Nowadays, brothers who want to keep their DL behavior on the low can make connections via ICP cameras and phone-sex lines, or find out where the meeting spots are where they can get as much sex as they can handle. The sky is truly the limit when it comes to finding men for sex, all thanks to the Web.

If you want to find out if your man has been making DL connections online, all you have to do is view the web-browser history information. Experienced DL men, determined to keep their activity undercover, have discovered that to keep their activity away from the house it is best to go to a local Internet café or Kinko's where they can get access to the Net. Many can go to friends' houses and cruise the Net. Many men have friends who are part of the club, and they cover for one another and provide an outlet to have sex or make connections outside of the home.

A computer software–designer friend recently told me about new software that can be installed on computers to record what you type, where you go, what you are looking for, and even capture screenshots of your computer, and you would never know that your activities are being tracked. This online "spy" is being used by people who want and need to know what their mates are doing online. He also informed me that there are even ways that you can have your mate's voicemail secretly forwarded to another phone. He told me he had this spyware installed on his home computer and found out that his partner was cheating on him.

I mentioned in an earlier chapter that when women get nosy they can find out a lot about their partner. Forget tracking down your man's online activities, just use the old-fashioned "I'm going to get in your business" attitude, and you will find out everything you need to know.

A DL friend of mine shared a story of how he got busted. His girlfriend had spent the night at his apartment, which she did on the weekends. After they had made love, she fell asleep. He said he couldn't sleep, so he got up and logged online to check his e-mail and to visit a couple of DL chat rooms that he enjoyed. For about thirty minutes he chatted back and forth with a brother who was trying to get him to come over to his apartment. He had told the brother that he would try and get away on Sunday night, after his girl had gone home. He would come over on his way from dropping her off.

When he went to get something to drink out of the kitchen, she woke up, and for some reason started looking at his laptop and reading the chat he had been having in the chat room. When he walked back into the bedroom, he was met with her screaming, "You fucking faggot!" He remembered just standing in shock while she grabbed her clothes, saying that she didn't believe this was happening to her. He tried to calm her down and get her to listen to him. He didn't know what to say, and he felt like someone had knocked the breath out of him. He just stood there with sweat popping out of his forehead. She picked up her cell phone and called someone to tell him or her that she was with a faggot. All he did was just stand there in shock. All he could think about was whom she was going to tell. He wasn't thinking about her, her hurt and pain, just about what this was going to do to his reputation.

I am amazed at how many brothers will go to adult bookstores and public parks to get a quick sexual fix. In every major city there is at least one well-known park where men meet in the dark, out of the public view, and have sex. No names exchanged, no conversation, just a look, a nod, or a " 'S'up" is all it takes.

I have attended family reunions held in a public park, and while the family was sharing baked beans, BBQ, and catching up, a few feet away on the walking paths men are making contacts with men. It can be done in less than five minutes. Before the family can pass the chicken, a sexual conquest can take place.

A friend from Louisville, Kentucky, told me that he was hanging out in Piedmont Park in Atlanta while attending a conference at a downtown hotel. He and a friend were walking through the park during the lunch break, and they saw a brother with a wedding ring having sex with another man.

In cities around the country, I have spent time at popular adult bookstores that are frequented by married men. They stop by on their way to work or on their way home from work. It is an easy process; in and out, pull it out.

DL connections are sometimes made without any thought of what you could be exposed to. There is no thought that goes into getting an STD, or being robbed, or getting busted by police. The need and strong desire to make that connection overrides all common sense. I have never seen any safe-sex posters, brochures, or messages that warn about HIV/AIDS in any of the places I have visited. I have never asked my trick if he had syphilis, herpes, HIV, or anything. If he looked good, or was the only brother at the spot, then he was the lucky one.

Women don't know if their man has made a stop at the bookstore, the Internet café, or the local cruise park when he walks in the door. It is up to the man to take responsibility and protect himself when active in these high-risk activities. A DL man has to think about what he has at home, who he will be going to bed with that night, and the love and support of his wife or lady. Sometimes the guilt is so heavy that, in his quiet time, it forces him to come out of denial and face reality. And that reality sometimes is more than he can handle. When I realized what I had done to my wife or to the women in my life, it made me cry and become very angry with myself. It was in those quiet times that I hated myself.

15

A NEED TO PROTECT OURSELVES AND OTHERS

D
r. Roland Tillard is an old-school Mature DL
Brother whom I met by placing an ad on a
popular Web site that caters to both DL and
gay men. I learned from our exchanging e-mails that he was
thirty-nine, married, and had several children still at home.
He was the music director of his church, and he was on the
faculty of the university in his hometown of Indianapolis.
He told me he was going to be in Chicago to attend a conference, and wanted to meet me. He was going to be traveling
without his family, but he would be with co-workers and the
choir.

We planned on meeting at his hotel room as soon as
he could get away from the preconference activities. When I
arrived at the hotel I called his room from the lobby. He gave

me his room number and asked me to come up. He answered the door with a smile and a firm handshake. He asked me to call him Doc. He was a very attractive brother. He wore his hair in shoulder-length locks and had on a pair of wire-framed glasses. We struck up a conversation about our families, work, and Chicago.

Twenty minutes into the conversation, I could tell he was ready to have sex. He kept looking at his watch, walking around the room, and fidgeting. I knew he had to meet with his chorus before their concert that night. So time was tight.

Finally he said to me, "You're a top, right?"

"Yeah, I'm always on top of my game," I said.

"Good, because I'm a bottom."

I changed the subject and started asking him more questions about his family. "Tell me about your children," I said.

He said he'd been married for ten years, had good children who were doing well in school, and his youngest was excited about a new bike he recently got. "I really want to be in a relationship with a brother," he said. "I'm hoping to find a brother I can have a tight relationship with."

He wanted more than just sex. He wanted a long-term committed relationship with a man, but he wanted to keep his wife, too. He explained that because he worked with a lot of white men, it would be easy for him to get a white lover, but he didn't want one. He wanted to be with a black man. Someone he could invite over for family functions and not have anybody question the "friendship."

I asked him, "Well, what do you think about me?"

"You're attractive, masculine, I could take you home to meet my wife and she would never suspect a thing," he said. "I'm comfortable with you. If the sex is good and we can vibe that way, you have excellent potential to be what I'm looking for."

After listening to all this, I started talking about his children again. I wanted to see how serious he was about going on with the sex. He had mentioned that it had been a long time since he'd had sex with a man. Sometimes long periods without sex will make men really aggressive. How much would he risk? I started talking about his little girl and found out that she played the piano. I could hear the pride in his voice when he talked about his little black princess. His oldest son played soccer, and the younger son was into basketball. He told me about their schools and how active he and his wife were in their education. He also told me that he had just bought a new house and now his wife wanted a new car.

But again he went back to what was on his mind. He was getting bored with my small talk.

"Look, bro, what about me and you stop talking so much and get busy," he said, looking frustrated.

ON THE DOWN LOW

"Cool," I said.

He went into the bathroom, came out with a towel wrapped around his waist, and got on the bed.

Again, I started up small talk. Anything to buy some time with him. I was giving him every opportunity to ask me about my life. He knew only what I had told him online, and most of that was made up.

He wasn't listening to me. His mind was elsewhere.

I asked him if he wanted to wait and get to know me better before we had sex, and said, "Let's hold off and do this later." I wanted him to realize that he could back out without any hard feelings. He didn't want to hear that. He wanted me. Not one time did he say a word about using condoms, or ask if I had one. He just positioned himself for the act that was to follow. He was ready to have sex with me, a stranger whom he had just met for the first time less than an hour ago.

Right before he thought that I was going to enter him, I stopped and said, "Look, man, I have to get out of here. I can't do this now, maybe later."

"What?! You got to go?!" he said.

"Maybe tonight or tomorrow we can hook up," I told him. "I'm really feeling you. I just can't do this right now."

"I want you to have this," he said.

"How long will you be in town?"

"Three days," he said.

"Okay, we'll hook up before you leave." But I had no intention of seeing him again.

Several months later I received an e-mail from him telling me that he had decided to tell his wife about his bisexuality. He was tired of hiding, creeping, and lying to himself and to his wife. He asked for my advice on how to have the conversation with her. He knew it would be difficult, but he was willing to deal with the consequences. He didn't want to continue to put his wife's life at risk. He wanted to tell her, come clean, and get on with his life.

I told him to write her a letter. Put it all on paper. Everything he wanted to tell her if he felt he could not talk to her. But I did tell him that if he wrote it out, it could backfire on him and she could use it in divorce court against him. He said he didn't care about that. He was willing to walk away from everything. All he wanted was to stay in the life of his children.

He did have that conversation with his wife. She cried, he cried, he told me. At the end of a very long night they agreed to try to work it out. She didn't want to leave him and she didn't want the children to grow up without a father in their lives. She felt that with counseling and prayer, they could get through this. She really felt that it was a temporary thing that he would grow out of. She blamed her recent weight gain and her need for material things. She was going to lean on God for strength and guidance.

Like a lot of men, he knew that this need was not going away. But he was willing to try to control it. He would try to talk to her when the need arose, to see if she could help him control this need.

Several weeks later he called me to tell me he was back on the Internet looking at pictures and making contacts with men. He still wanted to have sex with men, and he had not talked to his wife about it. He was going to try to fight the need by just looking at pictures, and making contacts. But he had no plans to make any steps toward having sex. Two weeks later, he called to tell me that he'd had sex with a man he met coming out of the mall, and that this man could be the right one for him, to meet his needs and allow him to stay with his family.

I placed an ad on another popular Web site to see how many brothers I could meet and how far I could take them. I received over two hundred hits over a sixty-day period. I chose five. One turned out to be a minister. We hooked up at my place. We didn't waste any time. Within fifteen minutes, he was in my bed.

He also didn't ask me to use a condom, nor did he bring one out. It was just like Dr. Tillard, and many others. My image and attitude were enough to make them have unprotected sex with me if I chose. Even when I stopped and told him that I didn't have any condoms, he said I didn't need one, that it was okay with him. We didn't have sex.

Some ads will allow you to tell what type of sex practice you are into. Safe or bareback. I have read many ads submitted by brothers who describe themselves as being bisexual, stating that bareback sex is their sex practice.

I talked to a twenty-nine-year-old brother from Baltimore who told me he was bisexual and HIV positive. He didn't consider himself as being down low. He loved women, and wanted to get married one day. But for now he was enjoying having sex with men. He said he would never date or be in a relationship with a woman while he was actively having sex with men. He thought that men who were on the DL were dogs. However, his unsafe sexual practice was putting the men he was with at risk of getting infected. I tried to get his justification for this behavior.

Many bisexual and gay men, black and white, do not use condoms. The reasons are all lame—they don't fit, they are too small, they don't feel right, you can't feel the skin, it takes too long to put on, it's going to break anyway, why put it on?

Or they don't want lose the opportunity to have sex. Or they are under the influence of drugs or alcohol. All excuses with consequences that can affect more than one person.

There have been many surveys conducted by health

departments, community-based organizations, and HIV-prevention agencies asking why condoms are not used by men who have sex with men. Many offer the above-listed reasons for why they don't use them.

The CDC has reported that there are 180,000 to 280,000 people who are HIV positive and don't know it because they have not taken the test.

All men who are having sex should protect themselves, regardless of sexual orientation. The facts speak loud and clear. I heard it said best this way: "This thing is real, it doesn't care anything about what you drive, work, live or how much money you have. The only thing that can be done to save yourself and anyone you are having sex with should be in your pocket, car, bedroom, or anyplace you can put it to make it accessible at all times. Do the right thing, save a life today." Don't get caught up and then have to deal with something that does not have a cure, something that will change your life forever. All it takes is you making the right choice, particularly if you are not going to give your women the choice.

My doctor once told me that she has HIV-positive judges, doctors, lawyers, and ministers. She said that in her private practice she has patients who are prominent black professionals, from age sixteen to one hundred. For the black community, HIV is still a taboo, and that secrecy hampers efforts by many to fight the spread of the disease.

16

NO MORE SECRETS

"Keep it on the down low, no one has to know."
—R. Kelly

Since beginning this work, I have received thousands of e-mails from women and men who are seeking answers to their questions about DL behavior, as well as from those who want to share their personal stories about experiences with a DL man. About 90 percent of the e-mail I receive is from women wanting answers to questions. On my Web site (www.livingdownlow.com) I list the top questions that I am asked, and which I have answered in this book. In addition, I now want to answer some questions not already covered. Please note that the responses given represent my personal opinions, the opinions shared by DL men who have participated in the focus groups I've conducted, and additional research that I've completed on the sexual lives of black men.

1. Why don't DL men just choose male sexual partners and stop pursuing relationships with women?

To understand the answer to this question, you have to delve into the psyche of the DL man. Many DL men aren't even remotely interested in establishing a relationship with a man. To these brothers, a sexual encounter with a man is a means of getting a quick sexual high, and that's it. From their perspective, relationships should be pursued only with women.

2. What is it about having sex with a man that DL men find appealing?

The reasons underlying the physical attraction between men vary among men. No single answer explains the attraction men have for one another. It's important for women who find that they are involved with a DL man to know that his sexual attraction to another man has nothing to do with her desirability as a woman. Many women have told me that they hope to "transform" their mates by increasing their sexual skill level, using sexual toys, and doing whatever is necessary to gain the sole sexual attention of their man. Frankly, those attempts are futile. A man engages in DL behavior because of what's going on in his mind and spirit. Any transformation of his sexual behavior can result only from changes inside him.

3. Why are secret sexual relationships between men called "down low," and is this behavior new?

Hidden sexual relationships between men have existed since the beginning of time. The heightened level of attention DL behavior is currently receiving is in response to the rising HIV infection rates among women. The phrase "down low" is a term borrowed from popular music where it is typically used to describe a love affair that must be kept top-secret, or "on the down low." Though the term originated in the heterosexual community, it has since been co-opted to describe the secret sexual encounters that occur between men.

4. Do white men live on the DL?

Yes. While the behavior may not be called "down low," secret sexual relationships happen between men in all parts of the world. There are men from all races, nationalities, and socioeconomic backgrounds who engage in the behavior. Recently I read that HIV infection rates are climbing in communities in Asia because of the increasing numbers of married men who are sexually involved with other men yet fail to disclose this information to their wives. They are living on the down low. Hopefully, as a result of this book, other communities will begin to explore the impact of this behavior as well. It should also be noted that there are women who live on the DL as well. But because their behavior does not impact HIV infection rates to the same degree, secret sexual relationships between women are not as widely discussed.

5. How did your coming clean about your DL behavior impact your children? What type of relationship do you have with your ex-wife?

As a father, the conversation about my former lifestyle was one of the most difficult that I've ever had to initiate with my children. I love them dearly and was fearful of hurting them. I was very concerned about how my disclosure might impact my relationship with them. Though getting through those conversations was not easy for any of us, we did. They have always remained supportive of me. Their love and respect for me as their father did not change. I trusted my children with the truth, and we have become closer as a result. My ex-wife and I have an excellent relationship. We have a mutual respect for each other as parents of our children. She has used the experience of having been married to a DL man to become a stronger woman, and uses her story to help other women. She is happily re-married, has a loving family, and is pursuing her life's passions.

6. If I'm married, how do I get my husband to wear a condom?

You begin by being as committed in your love for yourself as you are in your love for your husband. You have the right to feel safe and secure while enjoying sexual inti-macy with your mate. You can begin to negotiate condom usage by sharing your feelings and concerns openly and honestly. The conversation doesn't have to become a bat-tle over trust. It's important not to take an accusatory ap-proach. A defensive man is unlikely to set aside his feelings of hurt and confusion long enough to hear the concerns of his mate. Remember, not all men are on the DL. Your husband may interpret your request as an indi-cation that you are suspicious of him. Unless this is the case, take accusation and judgment out of the equation. Instead, share with your mate that condom use would help you feel a greater sense of physical and emotional se-curity. Explain to him that the safer you feel, the more of yourself you are able to share with him. Depending on the dynamics of the relationship, your mate may or may not be willing to use a condom. If not, you have to decide how you will respond. Remember that you control the terms by which you share sexual intimacy, and you have choices. Consult with your physician to explore the use of the female condom, or consider abstinence until he is persuaded to respond more positively to your concerns. If you are fearful that your husband is being unfaithful to you, make protecting yourself your number-one mandate: Insist on safety. A wounded ego can be healed. Many STDs aren't as easily overcome.

7. Why don't DL men just admit that they are homosexual and live openly as gays?

Many DL brothers don't consider themselves to be homosexual because their sexual attractions and encounters involve both same-sex and opposite-sex partners. In some instances, they identify as bisexual. What these men have in common with homosexual men is the severe negative stigma associated with homosexuality within the black community. Once labeled "homosexual," an individual is often ostracized from family and friends, despised by the broader community, and condemned to hell by the Church. Homophobia is rife in the black community. Many choose silence rather than carry the heaviness of guilt, shame, and judgment placed on the backs of those who openly identify as homosexual. Too often our community is afraid to talk about what's real. We pretend not to see what's right in front of us if it challenges the conventional social norms existing in our community. Reluctance to address those issues that make us the most uncomfortable has landed us where we are today. It's been a little over twenty years since AIDS was first identified, and as I write, the HIV virus disproportionately impacts black people the world over. Still, in the face of sickness and death, our community is disinclined to have the conversations that could save us. We have no realistic hope of protecting ourselves until we can talk about the attitudes and behaviors that contribute to our vulnerability.

8. Do you think homosexuality is learned behavior, or are you born that way?

Understanding the various pathways to sexual identity is a complex issue that even social and biological scientists debate. My personal belief is that each individual is born with a particular sexual orientation. Even though this predisposition exists, I also believe that social and environmental factors impact sexual identity. For example, there are individuals who report a shift in their sexual orientation from heterosexual to homosexual after situational rape or the trauma of sexual molestation. Similarly, there are individuals who report having relinquished homosexual behavior as the result of spiritual transformation. I suppose it's rather easy to see why the issue of sexual orientation and identity is the cause of such heated debate. My personal belief is that we are each born with a genetic predisposition, but that the social and emotional environment in which we live impacts the sexual identity that we eventually embrace.

9. Do you think that a DL man should be forgiven for his deceitful behavior once he admits it?

Yes, a DL man who comes to his mate in truth and accepts responsibility for his behavior should be forgiven. Forgiveness opens the door for healing and reconciliation, and is necessary if the relationship is to survive. As difficult as it may be to understand, most DL men don't engage in their closeted behaviors out of malicious intent. They don't want to live a double lifestyle and often don't understand it themselves. Many couples have been able to successfully restore their relationship by seeking professional help to sort through both DL behavior and its impact on the relationship. Though many black men are skeptical about the value of outside support, a good psychologist, spiritual counselor, or support group can be invaluable in helping to heal the emotional wounds resulting from this type of experience. Ideally, the two of you would engage in counseling as a couple. If you find that your mate is unwilling to get outside help, go without him. Be proactive in tending to your emotional health, and feel good about ensuring your physical and psychological well-being.

10. How do I tell my wife that I am bisexual and have been on the DL?

First, let me congratulate you on doing the right thing by honoring yourself and your wife with the truth. You've already taken the first courageous step by choosing to act in integrity with your wife. Think about what you want to say to her ahead of time, and know what you want as an outcome of the conversation. To help her prepare for the conversation, share beforehand that you have something difficult that you want to discuss, and set aside some uninterrupted time for the dialogue. Then, with as much honesty and compassion as you can muster, tell her about the internal battle you've been dealing with, and ask for her partnership and support in working through your struggle. Because you have been unfaithful to her, prepare yourself to apologize to her until she lets you know that she's heard it enough, and witnessed it in your actions enough to know that she can trust you again. The love that you share and the foundation that you've built together may result in her willingness to work through this with you. If not, you still must come to grips with your sexuality and seek professional counseling and/or guidance. Only when you are in integrity with yourself and with your wife will you find peace.

17

YOUR OPINION MATTERS

O ver the past three years there have been many stories done about the DL subject. And many more are to come. This issue is not going away anytime soon. It will be the subject of discussion on front porches, at club meetings, book clubs, discussion groups, conferences, and conventions. It will be debated, argued over, and people will walk away thinking that their opinion is the correct one. Enough said. I have never said that I have all the answers. I am not a professional HIV prevention specialist. I can only talk about my life and the research that I have conducted on the subject. When I first started on this journey, there was little or no information about DL men. Today, every major newspaper, television network, magazine, and your average Joe have talked about the DL from a position of authority. People will agree and disagree about what a DL man is. From the deep Bible Belt, where sex is not talked about outside of abstention, to the college campus where today's youths don't have the same opinions and hangups about sex as their parents, some have said that the DL doesn't even exist, that the whole issue was made up.

DL brothers on the East and West Coasts, DL brothers in the deep south and out west, all have the same behavior. There are DL men in all corners of our society. There is no place you can go where a DL brother will not be there. Since we know this, it is important that we continue to talk and listen.

I have received many e-mails from women and men, black and white, old and young, sharing their stories or feedback. I would like to share some of them with you. I have said that if you are talking about the issue, then it will have an impact on the behavior, and that is good conversation.

> I enjoy sex with both men and women. I like to fuck. I enjoy sex with women because there is no other penis involved. There is something about penetrating another man that really turns me on, I can't explain it. —Allen, Oakland

> I asked my husband if he knew anything about the down low community and he instantly replied yes. He got all moody and withdrawn and didn't talk

to me for the rest of the night. If he is on the DL, I am not out to hurt him. I want him to be happy, and be honest with himself, with or without me. I am just tired of the games. —Joyce, Atlanta

Black gay men have had many conversations about down low men. Many have had sex with them knowing that they were married, including me. I am not proud of this, but it happens every day. I applaud J. L. King and his work. He is doing more to bridge the gap between the black gay community and the black heterosexual community. —Max, Chicago

I am a homosexual man. I do not enjoy sex with women, but if a woman is attractive, I will take notice. I like and respect women. I like their feminine ways, the shape of their bodies, the way they walk and how they look at me if they find me attractive. I decided a long time ago not to engage in relationships of deceit and eventual heartbreak. I do not consider myself "gay" because I do not integrate the gay culture into my everyday life. I do not consider myself straight or bisexual because men who are primarily oriented to women generally use those terms. If I ever do use the term DL to describe myself, I use it for the sake of efficiency. Thanks for all you are doing to inform and educate our community. —Pete, Los Angeles

I think the continuing rise of HIV in the black community is ridiculous. Why would anyone knowingly put his or her partner at risk of being infected? I don't understand how we have the resources in our community; we test free in our community, yet the turnout is too sad to discuss. Are we in denial? Time changes and we must as black people change with the time. —Patricia, Houston

I work in a hospital. I started out as a Peer Health Educator and I have performed street outreach at places were youth congregate (i.e., parks, clubs, bathhouses, etc.). I have met Latina women who told me that they will have anal sex before having vaginal sex. Their fear is becoming an unwed mother. One twenty-three-year-old HIV-positive Latina woman was infected by her boyfriend. They only had anal sex. There are DL men in the Latino community and the rules are the same: Don't talk about it, and don't tell your women. —Darryl, Chicago

18

WOMEN STILL WANT A RELATIONSHIP

I spoke to a group of single, educated, successful, and beautiful sisters who emotionally expressed to me that they understood the risks of unprotected sex. They knew the facts about the transmission of HIV and other STDs. They knew that they could protect themselves from getting infected. That is not what was causing them to feel hurt and pain. What was causing them the deeper pain and hurt was the fear of not sharing their lives with a man who will love and respect them, a man who will honor the holy vows of marriage, a man whom they can trust. These sisters wanted the house in the 'burbs, the children, and the security of growing old with one man. They realized that they could provide two of the three, but they could not provide the man. They wanted answers about relationships. One sister wanted me to tell her how she is supposed to know if her potential soul mate is not on the DL, and what she and all of her sister friends are supposed to do to meet this need. She spoke with tears in her eyes about how she had done all the right things in her thirty-two years. She got an education, she had not had children out of marriage, she had excellent credit, she looked good, she went to church, and she gave back to her community. She said, "I'm tired of always being the bridesmaid, the big sister, the godmother, the aunt, the support system" to her married friends. She wanted a man and children of her own. What was she to do? She was scared and upset with brothers. She went on to say she didn't want to date outside of her race. A strong black father, who was her role model for the type of man she wanted to marry, had raised her. She didn't care if he was a blue-collar worker or CEO of a Fortune 500 company; she just wanted a man that would respect and love her.

When I hear these pleas from sisters, I have to ask myself what it is going to take to get DL men to realize that what they are doing is not right, and that their selfish attitude has a long-term effect beyond getting infected with HIV or an STD.

I learned the hard way how my actions can destroy

the spirit of a woman. I have experienced the pain that never goes away. If I could do it all over again, I would have fought my desires to cheat on my wife and on the women who have given me their love. I would have tried to communicate with my woman, and if I couldn't talk to her, I would have walked away—or I should have never have entered her life.

No woman deserves to be hurt by a man who is not honest and open with her about his desires. No man should make decisions for his woman that will impact her long after the relationship is over.

A majority of men are not on the DL. Men who are willing, able, and ready to be the type of man that women are looking for. Men who want to be with only one woman. Not with a man or with another woman, but with the woman whom he has promised to be with till death.

I encourage sisters not to give up on finding love. I encourage brothers to prove to women that they are not on the DL, and I beg brothers who *are* hiding their bisexuality to allow their women to decide if they want to be with them. Many sisters have told me that if they knew their man was bisexual they would be okay with that, because they would know going into the relationship who and what they were dealing with.

I hope, after this book has been read, that through my experiences, and the experiences of others that I have shared, both DL men and their women will be set free to live a life that is fulfilling and complete.

Acknowledgments

If you had told me two years ago that I would be a published author, I would have said you were crazy. There can be only one reason I am where I am today: God, who is the source of everything that I have become.

God has blessed me with the love and support of my children. Thank you for your unwavering faith in me and my dreams. I love you and pray that you will continue to be proud of me, especially after you read this book.

My father, Louis V. King, I hope you will understand the purpose of this book and allow me to do what God has directed me to do. Continue your powerful prayers that protect and guide me. I know that Ma is smiling at me from Heaven.

Brenda Stone King Browder, I pray my story helps you understand why I did what I did. I hope this heals the hurt and pain you have carried all these years. I know you will always have God's love for me, and for that I am truly blessed.

Marshall Douglas, my prayer partner, best friend, my brother, thank you for being "on one accord" with me and "touching and agreeing" with me—459 for life.

Juliet Dorris-Williams—my guardian angel who told me that while people would not like what I had to say, God would guide me—thank you for believing me.

Karen Hunter, this project is complete only because of you.

Debbie Cowell, my first editor, from day one you grabbed me by the balls and didn't let go until I let go of all the hidden stuff that I didn't want to share. Thanks, Debbie. I would also like to thank Janet Hill and Clarence Haynes at Broadway Books for all of their hard work to make this book one that's more than just about me and one that will change attitudes.

Alexis "Zo" Alexander, thank you for your vision. Thanks to Phil Wilson for giving me a national platform; to Tim Jackson for that first conversation in Austin, Texas; to Ako Kambon for telling me to listen to God and be obedient; to Mychal Wynn and Al "Coach" Powell for being my example of how to be a speaker who touches people.

Thank you to Wes Pullen for being there when it was just me and you, to Arnie Sutherland for your support and belief, and to Sherri Anderson-Elliott, the best personal banker a person can have. Thanks, Dr. Ron Simmons, for teaching me to understand black gay men; Callie Crossley, thanks for being my play big sister and my very first cheerleader; and thanks to Beth Vessel for pushing me to write, write, write.

Thank you, Ian Kleinert, my agent, for having contacts in the publishing industry who listened to you, and thanks to Manie Barron for knowing Ian. Thank you, Sharon Johnson, for writing an awesome proposal that paved the way for this book. James Morgan, thank you for being the first to plant the idea of writing a book; and Tim Moore, thanks for giving me your talent and time in the beginning.

Thank you, Black Entertainment Television (BET, especially Carol Green), Public Broadcasting Service, ABC News *20/20* (especially producer Melissa Cormick), and all the television networks, newspapers, magazines, and radio stations that mentioned me and my story.

Thanks to Delta Sigma Theta Sorority Inc. for your love, your support, and for being a leader in HIV education for women.

A special thanks to a few of the strong women who

shaped and molded me: Angie Tolliver, Debra Morehead, Angela Kenyetta, Peggy Nelms, Wilma Stone, Gail Stone Grant, Dorothy Stone Taylor Booker, Denise Duncan, and the many others I wish I could name. All of you taught me the power of the black woman.

I also want to give kudos to Lora Branch, Roslyn Harvey, Rae Lewis Thornton, Sandra Wimberly, and Virginia King, women I have met who are making a difference in their communities on HIV prevention and education.

E. Lynn Harris, you told me when I first met you in Cleveland in 2001 that I should get ready for where this message would take me. You said to stay strong. Your words of wisdom have paid off.

Lastly, to every person who has shared your story with me. I love you and I thank you for your prayers, support, and your love.